Recipes for Diabetics

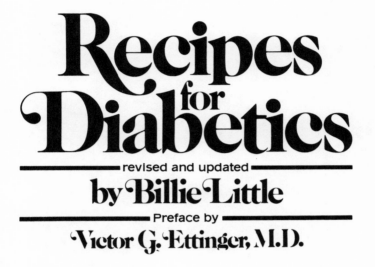

Recipes for Diabetics

revised and updated

by Billie Little

Preface by

Victor G. Ettinger, M.D.

A GD/PERIGEE BOOK

Perigee Books
are published by
The Putnam Publishing Group
200 Madison Avenue
New York, New York 10016

Library of Congress catalog card number: 80-84944
ISBN 0-399-50957-7

First Perigee printing, 1983
Two previous Grosset & Dunlap printings
Printed in the United States of America
1   2   3   4   5   6   7   8   9

CONTENTS

ACKNOWLEDGMENTS

So very many friends, relatives and diabetic patients have contributed their ideas and treasured recipes that we wish to give a special note of thanks to them and to the food companies, firms, newspapers and magazines whose information appears in this book. We gratefully acknowledge permission from the following:

Adolphs, 5355 Cartwright, North Hollywood, CA 91601

Alba Foods (skim milk products), 800 Third Ave., New York, NY 10020

Batter Lite Foods (fructose, Batter Lite cake batters, etc.), P.O. Box 321, Beloit, WI 53511

Beatrice Foods, 1526 South State St., Chicago, IL 69605

Borden, Inc. (Lite Line cheeses), 277 Park Ave., New York, NY 10017

Campbell Soup Company, 375 Memorial Ave., Camden, NJ 08101

Carnation Foods, 14th & Poplar, Oakland, CA 94607

Cumberland Packing Co. (Sweet 'n Low Division), 2 Cumberland St., Brooklyn, NY 11205. (Butter Buds), 1636 Taylor, Racine, WI. 53403

Diet & Health Products (Fisher Cheese Co.), P.O. Box 1886, Lima, OH 45802

Food and Nutrition Board, 2101 Constitution Ave., Washington, DC 20418

Frito-Lay, Inc., Exchange Park, P.O. Box 35034, Dallas, TX 75235

General Mills Chemicals, Inc., 4620 W. 77th St., Minneapolis, MN 55435. (Yoplait), P.O. Box 1113, Minneapolis, MN 55440

Good Food Unit #306, National Health Systems—The Times, P.O. Box 1501, Ann Arbor, MI 48106

Haddon House, Marlton Pike, Medford, NJ 08055

Henkel Corp. (dietary specialties), 4620 W. 7 St., Minneapolis, MN 55435

Knox Gelatin, Inc., 800 Sylvan Ave., Englewood Cliffs, NJ 07632

Kraft Foods, 500 Peshtigo Court, Chicago, IL 69690

Lever Brothers, New York, NY 10022

Tillie Lewis Foods, Inc. (low-calorie foods), P.O. Drawer J, Stockton, CA 95201

Eli Lilly & Company, Indianapolis, IN 46206

Thomas J. Lipton, Inc. (Wish-Bone Lite and other low-calorie salad dressings), 800 Sylvan Ave., Englewood Cliffs, NJ 07632

M C P Foods (Slim Set, mix for jams and jellies), P.O. Box 3633, Anaheim, CA 92803

National Dairy Council, 6300 North River Road, Rosemont, IL 60018

National Health Systems, P.O. Box 1501, Ann Arbor, MI 48106

Pillsbury Company (Sprinkle Sweet), 311 Second Street S.E., Minneapolis, MN 55414

Plough, Inc. (Ril Sweet), Memphis, TN 38101

Rosarita Products (low-calorie Mexican foods), Box 1427, 310 South Extension Road, Mesa, AZ 85201

Specialty Brands, Inc. (Spice Islands, Marie's Refrigerated Dressings), P.O. Box 2187, South San Francisco, CA 94080

Spreckels Sugar Co. (sugar products), 50 California St., San Francisco, CA 94111

Sterling Food Co. (soya, carob flour mix), 5118 Fourteenth Ave., N.W. Seattle, WA 98107

Sugar Lo (Parv-A-Zert, frozen dietetic desserts), 2001 Bacharach Blvd., Atlantic City, NJ 08401, Attn: Alan E. Kligerman

Superose Sweetener, G. H. Whitlock Process Co., P.O. Box 259, Springfield, IL 62705

Sweet 'n Natural (Sweet 'n Natural fruit sugar), P.O. Box 55086, Sherman Oaks, CA 91403; or P.O. Box 410, Brooklyn, NY 11202

Tropicana Products, Inc. (pure orange juice), P.O. Box 338, Bradenton, FL 33506

U.S. Government:

Department of Agriculture, Agricultural Research Service, Independence Ave., 12th & 14th St. S.W., Washington, DC 20251

Department of Agriculture, Science & Education Administration, Consumer & Food Economic Institute, Hyattsville, MD 20782

Department of Health and Human Services, Public Health Service, Food & Drug Administration, Consumer Communications Staff, 5600 Fishers Lane, HFJ, Rockville, MD 20857

SPECIAL THANKS TO: Miss Carol Edgar, Public Relations Division, Eli Lilly and Company, Indianapolis, IN, for her assistance and permission to use information contained in the many excellent booklets distributed by this fine company; to Mr. James R. Schmidt of Tillie Lewis; to the Public Health Service and other government sources; to Mary Helen Gunkler, R.D., Nutrition Department, General Mills, Inc.; and last but not least to Marie Slavens, our typist, for patiently wading through our notes.

Additional information on medication, reactions, travel and vacation, food care, and so on will be found in "Diabetes and You," available from the Superintendent of Documents, U.S. Government Printing Office, Washington, DC 20402. Also refer to the section on Printed Material Available at the back of this book for booklets, books, and other pertinent information that can be obtained for little or no charge.

FOREWORD

These recipes are intended to help and guide you in preparing and serving attractive, colorful, unusual, and satisfying meals while conforming to your diabetic diet.

It is important that you follow your doctor's diet orders explicitly and use only those recipes suited to your particular suggested calorie intake.

The variety of recipes offered is intended to stimulate your interest in following your diet strictly, proving that your diet need not be monotonous and unappetizing. Many of these recipes can also be enjoyed by the entire family.

DOCTOR'S PREFACE

Aretaeus of Cappadocia, in the first century A.D., wrote the first clinical description of diabetes mellitus, though it was known at least two millennia earlier. He described it as "a melting down of the flesh into the urine." *Diabetes* comes from the Greek verb meaning "to pass through," suggestive of the frequently large quantities of fluid taken in by mouth and put out as urine. *Mellitus* means "honey"; it describes the sweet taste of the urine from the glucose (sugar) it contains. This was discovered in Europe in the eighteenth century; however, physicians in India had been aware of it for centuries. The picture of a person melting away is ironic when we consider that the majority of people who have diabetes are not only *not* wasting but are substantially overweight, to the point of obesity.

Of what consequence is this disease? Between ten and twenty million people in the United States alone have diabetes, and as we become a fatter and less active society, the numbers are increasing at the phenomenal rate of 6 percent per year. Hardly an American family exists in which some relative is not afflicted. We all have several friends or acquaintances who have it. The economic burden is astronomical—$5.3 billion in 1975 (close to $10 billion in terms of our present devalued currency). And this figure is just the monetary cost; it doesn't count complications associated with diabetes. Nothing can quantify the awful toll in mental and physical suffering due to the ongoing depredations of this illness. Diabetes is now the leading cause of new blindness and is a prime contributor to death and disability from heart attack, stroke, kidney failure, and lower limb amputation because of gangrene. What a terrible price to pay, made even more disheartening because many of these problems are preventable!

We have learned much in the four thousand years since diabetes was first mentioned in Egyptian writings. Yet we find an ever increasing morbidity and mortality from it. Why? From my philosophical vantage point, it seems due to an "it can't happen to me" attitude. Any habit—be it smoking, overeating, overconsuming of alcohol—that interferes with our self-indulgence, in spite of the drawbacks, is ignored. More people—especially teenagers—are smoking more cigarettes now than ever before, in spite of the evidence associating this expensive habit with emphysema, lung cancer, heart attacks, and so on. Many people who develop diabetes are obese; not five or ten pounds too heavy, but twenty-five, fifty, a hundred, or even more. Is the medical community able to get the obese diabetic to work, and it most definitely is work, at saving his or her eyes, heart, legs? Silly question! "It can't happen to me!"

What exactly is diabetes mellitus? In very simple terms, it is the inability of the body to appropriately use the foods we eat. It is not one or two diseases with only a few causes. A multitude of factors are involved, some inherited, others environmental. Whatever the causes, 90 percent of diabetics can control the disorder by diet alone. Some may need additional help—injections of insulin, or pills that make the body use its own insulin more effectively. Physicians have known this for many years. Recently, we have also come to understand the very important effect of regular exercise in the treatment of most individuals with diabetes. Most people with the disease are older, overweight men and women. They have become less and less active, and spend more and more time watching and eating, instead of doing.

Diabetic people like this think that their disease will go away with a little pill or, horror of horrors, with a shot of insulin. Surprise, surprise, they are dead wrong. The pills do not work very well for most overweight diabetics; and insulin for them is ridiculous, because most obese diabetics have much larger amounts of insulin in their blood than would be needed if they were of normal weight. Their fatness prevents this overabundance of insulin from working. Why is this so? The cells of the body that normally respond to insulin have "protein handles" on their outside membrane. These handles are called *receptors*. Insulin attaches itself to the receptor, in some still-unclear way, and this allows these cells to take in an essential nutrient, glucose. Fat people do not have enough receptors. Somehow the pancreas, the manufacturing center for insulin, senses the effects of this decreased receptor number; it takes this as a signal to produce more insulin, which it releases into the blood stream. The insulin doesn't get to the cells because of the dearth of receptors; therefore more insulin is produced and the cycle is repeated. The number of receptors is inversely related to a person's weight.

How can someone with diabetes increase his or her receptors? It should be obvious to one and all that the first item on the agenda is weight loss. As the diabetic individual loses weight, the receptor number increases. This gives the insulin more places to attach, so the body cells can use the glucose they need. The blood glucose level is thus lowered.

Simple enough, one would think; cut down on food consumption (diet) and *voilà,* I am home free—no more high blood sugar, goodbye diabetes, so long blindness, and on and on. True enough, but we all know how hard it is to diet for several months, much less forever. It is boring when you are unable to eat all the goodies you want; and anyway, "it can't happen to me!" Well, Sir or Madam, it *can* happen to you, and it very likely will.

Dieting doesn't have to be hard or boring. Look through this book and you will find a lifetime supply of nutritious, nourishing, and satisfying recipes for the most demanding palate. Sit down to *three*—count them one, two, three—meals a day with recipes garnered from this culinary jewel and enjoy yourself. And instead of taking that between-meal snack, go for a brisk walk for at least twenty minutes. Not only will this help decrease your appetite, it will also burn up calories, improve your circulation, condition your muscle tone, and increase your own body's ability to burn up sugar. There is no magic in losing weight. Crash diets are just that; they all come crashing down in the long run.

I do not wish to slight the important role diet and exercise play in the therapy of those diabetics who have an absolute need for injections of insulin every day. These individuals will also benefit immeasurably from this book. New dining vistas will be opened for them as well, allowing greater variety in their daily fare. However, as mentioned previously, most diabetics are overweight and would not benefit much from insulin treatment as opposed to the mandatory need for weight loss. Be that as it may, this volume can admirably serve the needs of almost every diabetic, in conjunction with exercise and the avoidance of those substances which may produce unhappy end results.

Remember, you didn't become an obese person overnight, and you can't become a thin person that way either. Sitting around bemoaning this lack of a way to instant slenderness won't help. Get out there and gradually start building up your activity level to twenty, then thirty minutes every day, and when you come home fix yourself a glass of Apple Foam or a previously prepared Banana Freeze (see Index) and see how enjoyable and healthy and filling exercising and eating can be. Get out there and slim yourself to health and always, *always* remember: It could have happened to you but it didn't because you cared enough about yourself and your family to overcome each and every obstacle and emerge triumphant.

Good eating (but not too much)!

VICTOR G. ETTINGER, M.D.
Assistant Clinical Professor of Medicine
UCLA Medical School
Torrance, California

AUTHOR'S NOTE

I have written this book because many diabetics have expressed their desire for a cookbook with recipes and helpful suggestions specifically related to their dietary needs.

This collection offers a large variety of unusual and basic recipes that have been kitchen tested and used for hospital patients on diabetic diets. Any of these recipes may be adapted for general use by substituting the equivalent amount of regular sugar for the artificial non-caloric sugar substitutes. Where ingredients you are unable to tolerate are called for, you can usually omit them; the finished product may perhaps be a bit less tasty, but it can probably be eaten with enjoyment just the same.

The caloric content and the exchange-group breakdown for each measured individual serving have been carefully calculated. There are helpful hints for using diet ingredients, for restaurant dining, and for preparation of box lunches. We have also included reference materials—tables of weights and measures (including metric tables) weight tables, diabetic exchange lists (with a special table of packaged foods), tables of nutrient values of foods, aids to varying meals, and daily menu guides.

Cookbooks have been published to assist diabetics, but to my knowledge the subject has not been approached elsewhere from so comprehensive a point of view.

I had you all in mind while writing this, and I hope it will become the most useful book on your cookbook shelf.

Billie Little
(with appreciation to
Sally Murphy)

REMEMBER

that while many people (in addition to your doctor)—a dietitian or nurse, for example—can assist you in learning to control diabetes, it is up to *you* to:

1. Continue under medical supervision.
2. Use the exact amount and type of medication prescribed for you! Follow this plan, paying special attention to precise amounts and kinds of food and the time schedule prescribed for you by your doctor.
3. Use the exact diet plan worked out for you.
4. Do some exercise, in the same amounts, each day. (The latest information we have is that the right exercise helps produce the amount of insulin a diabetic needs. Consult your physician for *your* proper exercise program.)
5. In addition to your regular physical checkup, have a regular eye examination, *especially* if you are being treated with insulin; the American Association of Ophthalmologists reports that "about 12 percent of all new blindness in the United States is due to complications of diabetes."
6. Practice good habits of personal hygiene to minimize the possibility of infection.

WEIGHTS, MEASURES, AND THE METRIC SYSTEM

The homemaker who is planning meals for a diabetic needs to know something about food values. The following tables will help determine measurements for carbohydrates, fats, and proteins. Also included are equivalents for most of the measures used in these tables. Be sure to use standard measuring utensils, such as an 8-ounce measuring cup, tablespoon, teaspoon, and the like. (The dime stores also carry a set of measuring spoons covering sizes from 1/8 teaspoon to 1 tablespoon.) It is also a good idea to remeasure after cooking. There are a few foods that need not be measured; these are noted in the Exchange Lists.

EVERYDAY WEIGHTS AND MEASURES

3 teaspoons	1 tablespoon
2 tablespoons	1/8 cup
4 tablespoons	1/4 cup
5 tablespoons + 1 teaspoon	1/3 cup
8 tablespoons	1/2 cup
12 tablespoons	3/4 cup
16 tablespoons	1 cup
2 cups	1 pint
2 pints	1 quart
4 quarts	1 gallon
1 fluid ounce	12 tablespoons
16 ounces	1 pound
1 pound butter or margarine	4 sticks, 2 cups, or 64 pats or squares
1 stick butter	1/2 cup (approximate) or 16 pats or squares
Dash or "few grains"	up to 1/8 teaspoon

METRIC SYSTEM

Liquid Measure

The metric system is based on units of 10. For liquid measure, the simple metric unit is the liter, which is just a little larger than our quart. One teaspoon is equivalent to 5 milliliters (or 5 cubic centimeters—a unit that drug dispensers prefer).

Units of Measure

1 milliliter = 1 cubic centimeter
1000 milliliters = 1 liter

Equivalents

1 teaspoon = 5 milliliters
1 tablespoon = 15 milliliters
1 cup = 0.24 liter
1 pint = 0.47 liter
1 quart = 0.946 liter
1 gallon = 3.8 liters
1 fluid ounce = 29.57 milliliters

Unit Conversion

To convert	into	multiply by
gallons	liters	3.785
liters	gallons	0.264
liters	pints	2.113
quarts	liters	0.946

The boiling point of water is: 212.0° Fahrenheit, or 100° Celsius or Centigrade.

Dry Measure

The basic unit of metric weight is the gram; this unit is approximately one-thirtieth of an avoirdupois ounce and is mostly used in pharmaceutical and scientific work. The more convenient unit is the kilogram, weighing approximately 2.2 pounds.

Units of Measure

1000 milligrams = 1 gram
100 centigrams = 1 gram
1000 grams = 1 kilogram

Equivalents

1 ounce = 28.35 grams
1 pound = 0.45 kilograms
2.2 pounds = 1 kilogram

Unit Conversion

To convert	into	multiply by
grams	ounces	0.035
grams	pounds	0.002
ounces	grams	28.35
pounds	kilograms	0.454

Calories

1 gram carbohydrate . . . . . . .4 calories
1 gram fat . . . . .9 calories
1 gram protein . . . . .4 calories
1 cup nondairy whip . . . . . . .160 calories (approximately)
Examples: 1 teaspoon sugar is 5 grams carbohydrate (20 calories)
1 teaspoon margarine or butter is 5 grams fat (45 calories)

GENERAL RULES

MEASURING FOOD

Most foods should be measured. You will need a standard 8-ounce measuring cup, measuring teaspoon, and tablespoon, and an ounce or gram scale. All measurements are level. Most foods are measured after cooking.

Careful measurement is more important for meat and fat quantities than for fruit, juices, and starches. Careful measuring of vegetables is less important as they generally are low in calories and fat.

It is important to measure foods at the beginning so you become acquainted with real serving sizes. (However, it really isn't necessary for you to weigh every bean!)

FOOD PREPARATION

Meats may be baked, boiled, roasted or broiled (indoors or on outdoor grill). Do not fry foods except in fat exchange allowed for that meal. Vegetables may be prepared with the family meals, but the portion for the diabetic should be removed before extra fat exchanges or bread exchanges are added. Fat allowed in your diet may be used to season vegetables. Vegetables may be cooked in bouillon or fat-free meat broth if desired.

SPECIAL FOODS

It is not necessary to buy special foods. Select the diet from the same foods purchased for the rest of the family—milk, vegetables, bread, meats, fats, and fruit (fresh, dried, or canned without sugar). "Special dietetic foods" should be used with discretion; always check the labels of these foods for protein, carbohydrate, fat, and calorie content. Be sure additional calories in special diet foods are figured in the diet.

Note: Recent scientific tests indicate that saccharin may be dangerous to your health and may be cancer causing. A warning to that effect is now posted in stores where products containing saccharin are sold.

FREE FOODS

Seasonings: Cinnamon, celery salt, garlic, garlic salt, lemon, mustard, mint, nutmeg, parsley, pepper, sugarless sweeteners, spices, vanilla, and vinegar. *Other foods:* Coffee or tea (without sugar or cream), fat-free broth, bouillon, unflavored gelatin, sour or dill pickles, cranberries (with sweetener or sugar substitute).

FOODS TO AVOID

Sugars (cane/beet/raw/brown/Turbinado—all kinds), candy, honey, jam, jelly, marmalade, syrups, pie, cake, cookies, pastries, sweetened condensed milk, soft drinks, candy-coated gum; fried, scalloped or creamed foods; beer, wine and other alcoholic beverages.

EXCHANGE LISTS

Your registered dietitian or doctor will select items from the following food groups according to their carbohydrate, fat, and protein content, calorie count, and so on. To ensure good nutrition, your diet should include the same essential foods, sometimes referred to as the "basic six," recommended for everyone:

1. Milk
2. Vegetables
3. Fruits
4. Breads and Cereals (whole-grain, enriched, or restored), and Starchy Vegetables
5. Meat
6. Fat

Foods on the same list have about the same nutritional value. The groupings are called "exchange lists" because one food may be exchanged for another on the same list, *but* foods on one list may *not* be exchanged for foods on another list. Each diet plan includes foods from all exchange lists to give variety.

The diabetic on a rigid restricted-calorie diet should avoid too many bread, fat, and meat exchanges. The calorie counts and exchanges have been calculated from the diabetic exchange lists found on the next few pages. Different exchange groupings vary slightly. It is imperative that a diabetic follow the calorie prescription given him by the doctor and the exchange lists that are included with his or her own diet order. (A strict diabetic should recalculate these recipes if using a different exchange system.) Different methods of recipe preparation, interpretation of ingredients, types of non-nutritive sweeteners (both liquid and granulated), and so on, will vary the volume of the recipe and approximate yield. If the yield is different, the calories of the recipe need to be recalculated, and the exchanges refigured. (See page 19 for counting calories.)

EXCHANGE LISTS FOR MEAL PLANNING COURTESY OF THE AMERICAN DIABETES ASSOCIATION

(Excerpted from American Diabetes Association information prepared by Kathy Stols, R.D.)

An "exchange" is a measured *portion* of food. The size or quantity of each exchange on the list is already developed for you in easy household measurements.

One of the most important aspects of diabetes management is dietary care. The Food Exchanges are lists of foods grouped by similar values of carbohydrates, proteins, and fats so that one food can be substituted for another in your daily meal plans. Foods have been divided into six categories—milks, vegetables, fruits, breads, meats, and fats. Foods in any one group can be substituted or exchanged with other foods *within the same group*.

We suggest that you consult your physician or nutritionist about your meal plan. You will be told how many exchanges you can have from each of the six lists, taking into account how many calories will be best for you. The number of calories will be based on your health, energy needs, and physical activities.

Eat only those foods on the diet list. Eat only the amounts of food shown. Do not skip meals. Do not eat between meals.

List #1: Milk Exchanges:

One Exchange of Milk contains 12 grams of carbohydrate, 8 grams of protein, a trace of fat, and 80–90 calories.

NONFAT FORTIFIED MILK	quantity	calories
Skim or nonfat milk	1 cup	90
Powdered (nonfat, dry, before adding liquid)	1/3 cup	80
Canned, evaporated skim milk	1/2 cup	100
Buttermilk, *homemade* from skim milk	1 cup	90
Yogurt made from skim milk (plain, unflavored)	1 cup	90

LOW-FAT FORTIFIED MILK	quantity	calories
1% fat fortified (count 1/2 Fat Exchange)	1 cup	113
2% fat fortified milk (count 1 Fat Exchange)	1 cup	135
*Yogurt made from 2% fortified milk (plain, unflavored) (count 1 Fat Exchange)	1 cup	140
Sweet acidophilus	1 cup	140

WHOLE MILK	quantity	calories
Whole milk	1 cup	120
Canned, evaporated whole milk	1/2 cup	170
Buttermilk made from whole milk	1 cup	160
*Yogurt made from whole milk (plain, unflavored)	1 cup	120–140

*Commercial yogurt with cream added may have 200 or more calories (for plain; even more for fruit yogurt).

List #2: Vegetable Exchanges:

One Exchange of Vegetables contains about 5 grams of carbohydrate, 2 grams of protein, and 25 calories. One Exchange is 1/2 cup.

Asparagus	Greens:	Rhubarb
Bean sprouts	Beet	Rutabaga
Beets	Chards	Sauerkraut
Broccoli	Collards	String beans
Brussels sprouts	Dandelion	(green or yellow)
Cabbage	Kale	Summer squash
Carrots	Mustard	Tomatoes
Cauliflower	Spinach	Tomato juice
Celery	Turnip	Turnips
Cucumbers	Mushrooms	Vegetable juice
Eggplant	Okra	cocktail
Green pepper	Onions	Zucchini

The following raw vegetables may be used as desired:

Chicory	Lettuce
Chinese cabbage	Parsley
Endive	Radishes
Escarole	Watercress

Starchy vegetables are found in the Bread Exchange List.

List #3: Fruit Exchanges:

One Exchange of Fruit contains 10 grams of carbohydrate and 40 calories.

Note: Whole fresh fruits are an excellent source of fiber. (Fiber is an important component in the diet. Recent research indicates that including fiber in the diet can assist in controlling blood sugar.)

Apple	1 small	Applesauce	
Apple juice	1/3 cup	(unsweetened)	1/2 cup

Apricots, fresh	2 medium	Melon:	
Apricots, dried	4 halves	Cantaloupe	1/4 small
Banana	1/2 small	Honeydew	1/8 medium
Berries:		Watermelon	1 cup
Blackberries	1/2 cup	Nectarine	1 small
Blueberries	1/2 cup	Orange	1 small
Raspberries	1/2 cup	Orange juice	1/2 cup
Strawberries	3/4 cup	Papaya	3/4 cup
Cherries	10 large	Peach	1 medium
Cider	1/2 cup	Pear	1 small
Dates	2	Persimmon,	
Figs, fresh	1	native	1 medium
Figs, dried	1	Pineapple	1/2 cup
Grapefruit	1/2	Pineapple juice	1/3 cup
Grapefruit juice	1/2 cup	Plums	2 medium
Grapes	12	Prunes	2 medium
Grape juice	1/4 cup	Prune juice	1/4 cup
Mango	1/2 small	Raisins	2 tbsp.
		Tangerine	1 medium

Cranberries may be used as desired if no sugar is added.

List #4: Bread Exchanges:

One Exchange of Bread contains 15 grams of carbohydrate, 2 grams of protein, and 70 calories.

Note: Wherever possible, bread and cereal products should be whole grain. Fiber is an important component in the diet. Recent research indicates that including fiber in the diet can assist in controlling blood sugar.

Bread:		Biscuit (count 1 Fat	1
White (including French		Exchange)	
and Italian)	1 slice	Muffin, plain or fruit	1
Whole wheat	1 slice	(count 1 Fat Exchange)	
Rye or pumpernickel	1 slice	Plain roll, bread	1
Raisin	1 slice	Frankfurter roll	1/2
Bagel, small	1/2	Hamburger bun	1/2

Dried Bread crumbs   3 tbsp.

Tortilla, 6":   1
  corn (44 calories)
  flour (snack size)

Cereal:
  Bran Flakes   1/2 cup
  Granola   1/2 cup
  Other ready-to-eat   3/4 cup
    unsweetened
    cereal
  Puffed cereal   1 cup
    (unfrosted)
Cereal (cooked)   1/2 cup
Grits (cooked)   1/2 cup
Pasta (cooked)—   1/2 cup
  Noodles, Spaghetti,
  Macaroni
Popcorn (popped, no   3 cups
  fat added)
Cornmeal (dry)   2 tbsp.
Flour   2 1/2 tbsp.
Wheat Germ   1/4 cup

Crackers:
  Arrowroot   3
Crackers, round   5
  Butter-type (count
    1 Fat Exchange)
  Graham, 2½" sq.   2
  Matzoth, 4" × 6"   1/2
  Oyster   20
  Pretzels, 3⅛" long   25
    × ⅛" dia.
  Rye wafers, 2" × 3½"   3
  Saltines   6
  Soda, 2½" sq.   4

Dried Beans, Peas, and Lentils:
  Beans, Peas, and   1/2 cup
    Lentils (dried or cooked)

Baked beans, no   1/4 cup
  pork (canned)

Starchy Vegetables:
  Corn   1/2 cup
  Corn on cob   1 small
  Lima beans   1/2 cup
  Mixed vegetables   1/2 cup
  Parsnips   2/3 cup
  Peas, green   1/2 cup
    (canned or frozen)
  Potatoes, white   1 small
  Potatoes (mashed)   1/2 cup
  Pumpkin   3/4 cup
  Winter squash,   1/2 cup
    acorn, or
    butternut
  Yam or Sweet
    potato   1/4 cup

Prepared foods:
  Biscuit, 2" dia. (count   1
    1 Fat Exchange)
  Cornbread, 2" sq.   1
    (count 1 Fat Exchange)
  Corn muffin, 2" dia.   1
    (count 1 Fat Exchange)
  Potatoes, french-fried   8
    (count 1 Fat
    Exchange)
  Potato or Corn chips   15
    (count 2 Fat
    Exchanges)
  Pancake, 5" × ½"   1
    (count 1 Fat Exchange)
  Waffle, 5" × ½"   1
    (count 1 Fat Exchange)

List #5: Meat Exchanges:

LEAN MEAT: One Exchange of Lean Meat (1 oz.) contains 7 grams of protein, 3 grams of fat, and 55 calories.

Beef:	Baby beef (very lean), chipped beef, chuck, flank steak, round (bottom, top), all cuts rump, spare ribs, tripe	1 oz.
Lamb:	Leg, rib, sirloin, loin (roast and chops), shank, shoulder	1 oz.
Pork:	Leg (whole rump, center shank), ham, smoked (center slices)	1 oz.
Veal:	Leg, loin, rib, shank, shoulder, cutlets	1 oz.
Poultry:	Meat without skin of chicken, turkey, Cornish hen, guinea hen, pheasant	1 oz.
Fish:	Any fresh or frozen	1 oz.
	Canned salmon, tuna, mackerel, crab, or lobster	1/4 cup
	Clams, oysters, scallops, shrimp	5 whole or 1 oz.
	Sardines, drained	3
Cheese containing less than 5% butterfat		1 oz.
Cottage cheese, dry, 2% butterfat		1/4 cup
Dried beans and peas (count 1 Bread Exchange)		1/2 cup

MEDIUM-FAT MEAT: For each Exchange of Medium-Fat Meat count (add) 1/2 Fat Exchange. One ounce of Medium-Fat Meat provides 2 gm more fat than the lean meat.

Beef:	Ground (15% fat), corned beef (canned), rib eye, round (ground commercial)	1 oz.
Pork:	Loin (all cuts tenderloin), shoulder arm (picnic), shoulder blade, Boston butt, Canadian bacon, boiled ham	1 oz.
Liver, heart, kidney, and sweetbreads (note that these are high in cholesterol)		1 oz.
Cottage cheese, creamed		1/4 cup
Cheese: mozzarella, ricotta, farmer's cheese, Neufchâtel, Parmesan		3 tbsp.
Egg (high in cholesterol)		1
Peanut butter (count 2 additional Fat Exchanges)		2 tbsp.

HIGH-FAT MEAT: For each Exchange of High-Fat Meat count (add) 1 Fat Exchange.

Beef:	Brisket, corned beef (brisket), ground beef (more than 20% fat), hamburger (commercial), chuck (ground commercial), roasts (rib), steaks (club and rib)	1 oz.
Lamb:	Breast	1 oz.
Pork:	Spare ribs, loin (back ribs), pork (ground), country-style ham, deviled ham	1 oz.
Veal:	Breast	1 oz.
Poultry:	Capon, duck (domestic), goose	1 oz.
Cheese:	Cheddar types	1 oz.
Cold cuts		4¼″ × ⅛″ slice/1 1/2 oz.
Frankfurter		1 small

List #6: Fat Exchanges:

One Exchange of Fat contains 5 grams of fat and 45 calories.

POLYUNSATURATED		SATURATED	
Margarine, soft, tub or stick*	1 tsp.	Margarine, regular, stick	1 tsp.
Avocado (4″ dia.)**	1/8	Butter	1 tsp.
Oil: Corn, Cottonseed, Safflower, Soy, Sunflower	1 tsp.	Bacon fat	1 tsp.
		Bacon crisps	1 strip
		Cream, light	2 tbsp.
Oil: Olive**	1 tsp.	Cream, sour	2 tbsp.
Oil: Peanut**	1 tsp.	Cream, heavy	1 tbsp.
Olives**	5 small	Cream cheese	1 tbsp.
Almonds**	10 whole	French dressing***	1 tbsp.
		Mayonnaise-type Dressing	2 tbsp.

NON-DAIRY CREAMERS

Mocha Mix (40 calories)	2 tsp. (approximately)	
Powdered (33 calories)	1 tbsp.	″
Liquid (45 calories)	2 tbsp.	″

*Made with corn, cottonseed, safflower, soy, or sunflower oil only.

**Fat content is primarily monounsaturated.

***Can be used on fat-modified diet, if made with corn, cottonseed, safflower, soy, or sunflower oil.

NOTES ON SPECIAL
INGREDIENTS
USED IN RECIPES

1. In order to reduce the caloric content of numerous recipes without affecting quality, we have included various diet ingredients available in local supermarkets. We have calculated the calories and exchange groupings in our recipes using the following diet products:

    diet margarine
    diet mayonnaise
    diet salad dressings
    imitation dairy and nondairy products
    diet puddings
    diet sauces and toppings

    If you prefer to use an ingredient other than the diet supplement, you will have to adjust the calories and exchanges.

2. Sweeteners: No-calorie sweeteners may be substituted for sugar in many recipes, and also used on foods that need a certain amount of sweetening. They are sold in granulated, liquid, and tablet form. Granulated sweetener may be sprinkled on cereals and fresh fruits; it dissolves immediately. For cold beverages the liquid is most convenient, and either the tablet or the granulated form may be used in cooking or in hot beverages. For best results, add the sweetening agent toward the end of the cooking process, since the sweetening power is lessened when exposed to high or low temperatures for a long period of time.

    Sweeteners are available with either a calcium or a sodium base. Calcium-based sweeteners are slightly less sweet than the sodium forms. They are suggested for the diabetic who is on a low-sodium diet.

If you find too much substitute has been used, and that it leaves a bitter taste in the mouth, counteract it with a little salt (if it is permitted in your diet).

The many sugar substitutes on the market include Ril Sweet, saccharin, Sprinkle Sweet, Sucaryl, Sugartwin, Superose, Sweet and Light, Sweet Lite (Fructose), Sweet 'N, Sweet 'n Low, and Sweeta. There are also others, which you may prefer.

For *Substitute Sugar Syrup*, combine equal quantities of water and sugar substitute. Bring to a boil; boil 5 minutes or so. Store in a covered jar in your refrigerator and use for sweetening cold drinks. (This may be used in place of the commercial liquid sweetener.)

SYRUPS: (May be used to sweeten fruits for canning.)

Light: 7 teaspoons of sugar substitute and 4 cups of water. Boil together 5 minutes. Skim. Makes 4 1/2 cups.

Medium: 13 teaspoons substitute, 3 cups water. Boil 5 minutes. Skim. Makes approximately 3 cups.

Heavy: 20 teaspoons substitute, 2 cups water. Boil 5 minutes. Skim. Makes 2 2/3 cups.

GLAZES: Non-nutritive sweetener equivalent to 1 cup brown sugar; juice and grated rind of 1 orange.

Non-nutritive sweetener equivalent to 1 cup sugar; 1/2 cup cider, dietetic maraschino cherry juice, or sweet pickle juice.

1/2 cup (4 ounces) dietetic currant jelly, melted.

1/2 cup dietetic orange marmalade, softened.

There are several brown sugar substitutes available, but if you cannot locate any and brown sugar is called for in a recipe, put granulated white sugar substitute in a frying pay over *very low heat;* stir constantly until caramelized.

Use bulk non-nutritives for baked goods, such as cakes, cookies, bread. For drinks, use liquid non-nutritive sweeteners.

Liquid sweeteners are used by the drop. For example: 1/2 cup of granulated regular sugar, or granulated sugar substitute, is the equivalent of 1 tablespoon of liquid sweetener.

3. All diet margarines contain fewer than half the calories of regular margarine—17 calories per teaspoon, 50 calories per tablespoon. Although diet margarine is not recommended for frying, it can, with proper care, be used (first melt *slowly* in a frying pan; add food, cover, and cook over *low* heat). When baking, remember that it has only half the fat content of regular margarine; so, since tampering with the fat content of baked goods can ruin the finished products, we suggest using the regular soft-form or stick-form margarines in recipes calling for more than two tablespoons of margarine.

4. WINE AND LIQUOR NOTES. The recipes containing alcohol are not for diabetics without explicit consent of their own doctor. Each recipe containing beer, liquers, liquor, or wine is specially marked.

5. PURE ORANGE JUICE NOTE. Remember that pure orange juice contains approximately 11–12 percent natural fruit sugars; consult your physician about using it.

AIDS TO VARYING MEALS

Bake, broil, or roast meats. Bake, broil, or poach fish.

Add herbs to meat and vegetables. Use 1/4 teaspoon dry herbs for each 6 servings of fish, meat, or vegetables. Try basil, rosemary, garlic salt, dry mustard, or curry powder with beef or lamb; rosemary or savory with chicken, fish, or veal. Season tomatoes with curry powder, basil, or oregano; turnips with rosemary; cabbage with savory; zucchini or carrots with thyme or nutmeg; cauliflower with dill; spinach with marjoram or nutmeg.

The addition of seasoning salt and lemon pepper to recipes gives an entirely new taste.

To enhance dishes use a variety of condiments in lieu of salt: Chervil for soups and eggs (1/2 teaspoon for 4 servings); Beau Monde for eggs, fish, meats, sauces, and stuffing (1/2 teaspoon for 4 servings). Mei Yen in shrimp soufflé (1 1/2 teaspoons) or 1 tablespoon to either 4 eggs or 3 cups milk in other soufflés. Bay leaf, celery salt, or marjoram (1 teaspoon to 1 teaspoon salt) for stews. Green onion seasoning (1 teaspoon to 4- to 6-pound chicken). Tarragon (2 teaspoons to 4- to 6-pound chicken) for stuffing. (Note: Beau Monde and Mei Yen are salt substitute condiments which contain traces of salt and sugar, and should, therefore, be used sparingly.)

Add herbs and spices to liquids. Be sure you thoroughly crush any whole spice or leaves—such as anise seed, basil, bay leaf, oregano, rosemary, thyme—or if left whole—such as bay leaf or cinnamon stick—remove before serving.

Interesting meals may be prepared if you are careful in selecting from your Exchange Lists. For instance, you may prepare a stew if you select one small potato from the Bread Exchange (List 4) and add

34

vegetables and meat according to your own meal plan; or you might wish to have a spaghetti dinner by using spaghetti from Bread Exchange (List 4), cheese from Meat Exchange (List 5), and meat sauce.

Soy margarine or Soyamaise is a good substitute for margarine or butter; both have less fat content (if you are able to tolerate soy derivatives).

Use non-dairy whips. Each cup averages about 160 caloires. Note: Watch for coconut and palm oil, because coconut and palm oils are saturated fats.

Good sauces may be made from commercial sweet-and-sour barbecue sauce or teriyaki barbecue marinade—but be sure to check the sugar content.

Low-calorie diet spreads are available and may be used for sandwiches, hors d'oeuvres, and so on.

Unusual low-calorie or water-packed fruits, such as bing cherries, fruits for salads, Kadota figs, mandarin oranges, pineapple spears, and purple plums, are also available.

ADDITIONAL SUGGESTIONS

Measure dry ingredients before liquid; this will save washing utensils!

Sift flour *before* you measure when the recipe calls for sifted flour. Sift the flour into a bowl or onto a sheet of waxed paper, then spoon into measuring utensil. Level with a spatula or knife.

Molasses or syrup flows more easily if measuring utensil is rinsed in cold water and then lightly greased.

1 medium egg = 1/4 cup eggs.

Have eggs at room temperature.

Arrowroot: 1 tablespoon = 1 Bread Exchange. (May be used to thicken fruit juice so juice can be used as spread.) Arrowroot powder may be used in place of flour; use half as much arrowroot as flour. In recipes which use arrowroot, flour may also be used, but be sure to double the amount.

Cornstarch: 2 tablespoons = 1 Bread Exchange. May be used to thicken fruit juice for use as spread.

Egg Yolk: 1 egg yolk = 1 Fat Exchange. Use in place of 1 tablespoon flour for thickening liquids. (Yields 3 grams protein, 5 grams fat, 300 grams cholesterol, and no carbohydrate. Note: Egg yolks are of different food value than flour and are high in cholesterol.)

Flour (all-purpose, sifted): 1 tablespoon = 1/3 Bread Exchange. 2 1/2 tablespoons = 1 Bread Exchange.

Tapioca: 1 teaspoon, no Exchange necessary. (This is used mostly for sweet sauces. In thickening power this is equivalent to 1 tablespoon flour.)

The following items are on the market and readily available:

Nondairy whipped topping (D-Zerta,
    Dream Whip) ....1 tablespoon = 8 calories
    (can be found on the dessert shelf)
Nondairy whipped topping (Cool
    Whip) ....1 tablespoon = 14 calories
    (can be found in the frozen food section)
Diet gelatin (D-Zerta) ....1/2 cup = 8 calories
    (can be found on the dessert shelf)
Diet margarine (Imperial, Weight
    Watchers) ....1 tablespoon = 50 calories
    (can be found in the refrigerator section)
Sour half-and-half* ....1 cup = 160 calories
    (can sometimes be found in refrigerator section)
Imitation sour cream (Imo) ......1 cup = 304
(Note: This contains saturated fat, coconut and/or palm oil, and
therefore should be used sparingly.)

*Sour half-and-half can also be made using 1 cup half-and-half and 1 tablespoon vinegar or lemon juice.

EATING OUT

Suggestions For Restaurant Dining
And For Preparing Lunches To Be
Eaten Away From Home

The question most frequently asked by people on diabetic diets is "How do I make this diet fit my normal, daily routine?" This is extremely important both to children and adults. Size of portions will depend on individual calorie requirements and allowed food exchanges.

LUNCH-BOX MEALS

1. Bread Exchange: use either bread or crackers.
2. Fat Exchange: butter or mayonnaise; cream for beverages.
3. Fruit Exchange: use fresh fruit, unsweetened canned fruits, or fruit juices.
4. Meat Exchange: hard-boiled eggs, cold cuts, roast beef, turkey, chicken, ham, cheese, cottage cheese, peanut butter.
5. Milk Exchange: as beverage.
6. Vegetable Exchange: raw vegetables such as carrots, celery, cherry tomatoes, cucumber sticks, green pepper rings, radishes, whole tomatoes.
7. Yogurt: non-fat. (Note: Watch sugar in fruit yogurt.)

LUNCH-BOX SUGGESTIONS

SANDWICH: Composed of Bread Exchange (1 or 2 slices of bread), Meat Exchange (turkey or beef), Fat Exchange (butter or mayonnaise), and lettuce, sliced tomato, or other vegetable.

SANDWICH FILLINGS: for people on high-calorie diets, use chicken, egg, or tuna salad, for example.

SNACKS: graham crackers and butter
cheese and crackers
peanut butter and crackers
crackers and cold cuts, fish, or poultry

Examples

Milk (Thermos or purchased at school)
Sandwich of turkey or peanut butter
Fresh fruit—apple or tangerine
Carrot and celery sticks

Sandwich or cheese and crackers or cottage cheese
Fresh fruit—pear
Fresh tomato
Coffee with cream, or milk
Yogurt (see note, p. 25)

HOT LUNCH PROGRAMS

Straight meat entrée with vegetables or plain hamburger sandwich or plain hot dog on a bun
Fresh fruit
Salad with controlled diet dressing
Beverage—water, milk, coffee, or tea

Assortment from List 2: raw vegetable as desired, without sauces
Cold baked chicken
Bread and butter
Fresh fruit
Milk or hot beverage, as desired

DINING OUT HINTS

It can be easy to dine out comfortably on your calorie-restricted diet if you keep your exchange groupings in mind. Avoid dishes you are unsure of, such as casseroles, creamed foods, and other dishes that might have "hidden" ingredients.

1. Order plain soups, such as consommé, French onion, vegetable.

2. When ordering a salad, ask for your dressing "on the side" so you can measure the amount according to the fat exchanges you are allowed for that meal. If your fat exchanges are limited, a lemon wedge or vinegar (wine or cider) is usually available upon request.

   Sliced tomatoes are usually available upon request. Order them without dressing or with the dressing on the side.

3. In selecting entrées, choose meat items that are either baked, broiled, poached, or roasted. Ask the restaurant to eliminate butter from their preparation. The following are recommended:
   a. Baked or broiled chicken.
   b. Broiled shish-kabob or brochette without marinade.
   c. Broiled or baked seafood or fish.
   d. Broiled steak.
   e. Hamburger steak.
   f. Prime rib, roast beef.
   g. Roast turkey (account for dressing and gravy in appropriate food groups).

   Request that sauces and gravies be eliminated from your entrée or brought separately.

4. Order hot and cold cereals plain. Use milk or cream on cereals according to your exchange pattern.

5. Order bread or rolls without fat, according to your exchange pattern. Order toast dry.

6. Plain potatoes are readily available, either baked or boiled. For oven-browned or mashed potato, figure one bread exchange plus one fat exchange.

7. Order cooked vegetables plain; if not available, figure one extra fat exchange per serving of vegetables.

8. Recommended vegetables commonly served in restaurants include green beans, tomatoes, carrots, peas, corn on the cob, mixed vegetables, asparagus.

9. Order eggs poached or soft cooked; for fried or scrambled eggs, if prepared in a skillet, add one fat exchange.

10. Order bacon or sausage crisp.*

11. Fresh fruit is usually available (in season); choose banana, half grapefruit (plain), melon wedge, or fresh strawberries. Stewed prunes are often available without sugar syrup.

12. Order unsweetened fruit juice, or fresh fruit juice.

13. Order yogurt (plain) in lieu of sour cream.

*Nonetheless, these are still fats and should be considered as such.

DAILY MENU GUIDE

Eat your meals at about the same time every day. Eat only the amounts given on your diet plan and do not skip meals.

Use of the exchange lists is based on the recommendations of the American Diabetes Association and The American Dietetic Association in cooperation with the National Institute of Arthritis, Metabolism, and Digestive Diseases and the National Heart and Lung Institute of the U.S. Public Health Service, Department of Health and Human Services.

Since an adequate understanding of this diet is essential to its proper use, consultation with a professional (preferably a physician, dietition, or nurse) is recommended at the time you are given the diet and at regular intervals as needed. For additional information on diabetic diets, "Exchange Lists for Meal Planning" may be purchased for fifty cents from the American Diabetes Association, 2 Park Avenue, New York, NY 10016.

INSTRUCTIONS FOR DAILY MENU GUIDE

The foods allowed in your diet should be selected from the exchange lists. Menus should be planned on the basis of the daily menu guide. Foods in the same list are interchangeable because, in the quantities specified, they provide approximately the same amounts of carbohydrate, protein, and fat. For example, when our menu calls for one Bread Exchange, any item in List 4 may be used in the amount stated. If two Bread Exchanges are allowed, double the specified amount of one item or use one Exchange of each of *two* foods in List 4. A day's sample menus are given to illustrate correct use of the exchange lists.

CALORIE DIETS

The following suggested diets include a breakdown of exchange lists for breakfast, lunch, and dinner.

1000 Calories (approximately) carbohydrate . . . . . . .130 gm
protein . . . . .55 gm
fat . . . . .30 gm

Breakfast

1 1/2 Fruit Exchanges (List 3)
2 Bread Exchanges (List 4)

1 Fat Exchange (List 6)
1/2 cup nonfat milk (List 1)

Breakfast (Example)

Orange juice . . . . .3/4 cup
Toast . . . . .1 slice
Cereal, dry . . . . .3/4 cup
Margarine . . . . .1 tsp.
Nonfat milk . . . . .1/2 cup

Lunch

2 Meat Exchanges (List 5)

1 Bread Exchange (List 4)
Vegetable(s) as desired (List 2)
1 Fruit Exchange (List 3)
1/2 cup nonfat milk (List 1)

Lunch (Example)

Cheese . . . . .2 1-oz.
slices
Bread . . . . .1 slice
Dill pickles, radishes as desired
Apple . . . . .1 small
Nonfat milk . . . . .1/2 cup
Mustard . . . . .as desired

Dinner

2 Meat Exchanges (List 5)
1 Bread Exchange (List 4)
1 Vegetable Exchange (List 2)
Vegetable(s) as desired (List 2)
1 1/2 Fruit Exchanges (List 3)
1 Fat Exchange (List 6)
1/2 cup nonfat milk (List 1)

Dinner (Example)

Chicken, baked . . . . . .2 oz.
Peas . . . . .1/2 cup
Tomatoes . . . . .1/2 cup
Lettuce, endive . . . . . . .as desired
Fruit cocktail . . . . . . .3/4 cup
Margarine . . . . .1 tsp.
Nonfat milk . . . . .1/2 cup

Bedtime Feeding

1/2 Bread Exchange (List 4)
1/2 cup nonfat milk (List 1)

Bedtime Feeding (Example)

Graham cracker . . . . . .1 square
Nonfat milk . . . . .1/2 cup

1200 Calories (approximately)

carbohydrate . . . . . . .145 gm
protein . . . . .65 gm
fat . . . . .40 gm

Breakfast

1 1/2 Fruit Exchanges (List 3)
1 Bread Exchange (List 4)
1 Meat Exchange (List 5)
1 Fat Exchange (List 6)
1 cup nonfat milk (List 1)

Breakfast (Example)

Orange juice . . . . .3/4 cup
Toast . . . . .1 slice
Egg 1
Margarine . . . . .1 tsp.
Nonfat milk . . . . .1 cup

Lunch

2 Meat Exchanges (List 5)

2 Bread Exchanges (List 4)

1 Vegetable Exchange (List 2)
1 Fruit Exchange (List 3)
1 Fat Exchange (List 6)
1/2 cup nonfat milk (List 1)

Lunch (Example)

Cheese . . . . .2 1-oz.
                                       slices
Beef bouillon . . . . .as desired
Bread . . . . .1 slice
Saltine crackers 6
Carrot and celery sticks 1/2 cup
Apple . . . . .1 small
Margarine . . . . .1 tsp.
Nonfat milk . . . . .1/2 cup
Mustard . . . . .as desired

Dinner

2 Meat Exchanges (List 5)
1 Bread Exchange (List 4)
1 Vegetable Exchange (List 2)
Vegetable(s) as desired (List 2)
1 Fruit Exchange (List 3)
1 Fat Exchange (List 6)

Dinner (Example)

Chicken, baked . . . . . .2 oz.
Potatoes, mashed . . . . .1/2 cup
Tomatoes . . . . .1/2 cup
Lettuce, radishes . . . . .as desired
Fruit cocktail . . . . .1/2 cup
Margarine . . . . .1 tsp.

Bedtime Feeding

1 Bread Exchange (List 4)
1/2 cup nonfat milk (List 1)

Bedtime Feeding (Example)

Graham crackers . . . . .2 squares
Nonfat milk . . . . .1/2 cup

1500 Calories (approximately)

carbohydrate . . . . . . .195 gm
protein . . . . .75 gm
fat . . . . .50 gm

Breakfast

2 Fruit Exchanges (List 3)
2 Bread Exchanges (List 4)

1 Meat Exchange (List 5)
1 Fat Exchange (List 6)
1 cup nonfat milk (List 1)

Breakfast (Example)

Orange juice . . . . .1 cup
Cereal, dry . . . . .3/4 cup
Toast . . . . .1 slice
Egg 1
Margarine . . . . .1 tsp.
Nonfat milk . . . . .1 cup

Lunch

3 Meat Exchanges (List 5)

2 Bread Exchanges (List 4)
1 Vegetable Exchange (List 2)
2 Fruit Exchanges (List 3)
1 Fat Exchange (List 6)

Lunch (Example)

Cheese . . . . .3 1-oz.
                                 slices
Bread . . . . .2 slices
Carrot and celery sticks 1/2 cup
Apples . . . . .2 small
Mayonnaise-type
    dressing . . . . .2 tsp.

Dinner

3 Meat Exchanges (List 5)
2 Bread Exchanges (List 4)

2 Vegetable Exchanges (List 2)
Vegetable(s) as desired (List 2)
1 Fruit Exchange (List 3)
1 Fat Exchange (List 6)
1/2 cup nonfat milk (List 1)

Dinner (Example)

Chicken, baked . . . . . .3 oz.
Peas . . . . .1/2 cup
Potatoes, mashed . . . . .1/2 cup
Tomatoes . . . . .1 cup
Lettuce, chicory . . . . . .as desired
Fruit cocktail . . . . .1/2 cup
Margarine . . . . .1 tsp.
Nonfat milk . . . . .1/2 cup
French dressing,
    low-calorie . . . . .1 tbsp.

Bedtime Feeding

1 Bread Exchange (List 4)
1/2 cup nonfat milk (List 1)

Bedtime Feeding (Example)

Graham crackers . . . . .2 squares
Nonfat milk . . . . .1/2 cup

1800 Calories (approximately)

carbohydrate . . . . .225 gm
protein . . . . .90 gm
fat . . . . .60 gm

Breakfast

2 Fruit Exchanges (List 3)
2 Bread Exchanges (List 4)
1 Meat Exchange (List 5)
1 Fat Exchange (List 6)
1 cup nonfat milk (List 1)

Breakfast (Example)

Orange juice . . . . .1 cup
Toast . . . . .2 slices
Egg 1
Margarine . . . . .1 tsp.
Nonfat milk . . . . .1 cup

Lunch

2 Meat Exchanges (List 5)

2 Bread Exchanges (List 4)
1 Vegetable Exchange (List 2)
2 Fruit Exchanges (List 3)
2 Fat Exchanges (List 6)

Lunch (Example)

Cold cuts 1 1/2-oz
                              slice
Cheese . . . . .1 oz.
Bread . . . . .2 slices
Carrot and celery sticks 1/2 cup
Banana . . . . .1 small
Mayonnaise-type
    dressing . . . . .4 tsp.

Dinner

3 Meat Exchanges (List 5)
3 Bread Exchanges (List 4)

2 Vegetable Exchanges (List 2)
Vegetable(s) as desired (List 2)
1 Fruit Exchange (List 3)
2 Fat Exchanges (List 6)
1/2 cup nonfat milk (List 1)

Dinner (Example)

Chicken, baked . . . . . .3 oz.
Peas . . . . .1/2 cup
Potatoes, mashed . . . . .1/2 cup
Bread . . . . .1 slice
Tomatoes . . . . .1 cup
Lettuce, escarole . . . . .as desired
Fruit cocktail . . . . .1/2 cup
Margarine . . . . .2 tsp.
Nonfat milk . . . . .1/2 cup
French dressing,
    low-calorie . . . . .1 tbsp.

Bedtime Feeding

2 Bread Exchanges (List 4)
1 Meat Exchange (List 5)
1/2 cup nonfat milk (List 1)

Bedtime Feeding (Example)

Bread . . . . .2 slices
Roast beef, lean . . . . . .1 oz.
Nonfat milk . . . . .1/2 cup
Mustard . . . . .as desired

2000 Calories (approximately)

carbohydrate . . . . . . .245 gm
protein . . . . .110 gm
fat . . . . .65 gm

Breakfast

2 Fruit Exchanges (List 3)
2 Bread Exchanges (List 4)

1 Meat Exchange (List 5)
2 Fat Exchanges (List 6)

1 cup nonfat milk (List 1)

Breakfast (Example)

Orange juice . . . . .1 cup
Cereal, dry . . . . .3/4 cup
Toast . . . . .1 slice
Egg 1
Bacon, crisp . . . . .1 slice
Margarine . . . . .1 tsp.
Nonfat milk . . . . .1 cup

Lunch

3 Meat Exchanges (List 5)

2 Bread Exchanges (List 4)
Vegetable(s) as desired (List 2)
1 Vegetable Exchange (List 2)
2 Fruit Exchanges (List 3)
1 Fat Exchange (List 6)

1 cup nonfat milk (List 1)

Lunch (Example)

Cold cuts . . . . .two 1 1/2-oz.
                                              slices
Cheese . . . . .1 oz.
Bread . . . . .2 slices
Dill pickles, radishes . .as desired
Carrot and celery sticks 1/2 cup
Apples . . . . .2 small
Mayonnaise-type
    dressing . . . . .2 tsp.
Nonfat milk . . . . .1 cup

Dinner

3 Meat Exchanges (List 5)
3 Bread Exchanges (List 4)

2 Vegetable Exchanges (List 2)
Vegetable(s) as desired (List 2)
1 Fruit Exchange (List 3)
1 Fat Exchange (List 6)
1 cup nonfat milk (List 1)

Dinner (Example)

Chicken, baked . . . . . .3 oz.
Peas . . . . .1/2 cup
Potatoes, mashed . . . . .1/2 cup
Bread . . . . .1 slice
Tomatoes . . . . .1 cup
Lettuce, etc. . . . . .as desired
Fruit cocktail . . . . . . .1/2 cup
Margarine . . . . .1 tsp.
Nonfat milk . . . . .1 cup
French dressing,
    low-calorie . . . . .1 tbsp.

Bedtime Feeding

2 Bread Exchanges (List 4)
2 Meat Exchanges (List 5)
1 Fruit Exchange (List 3)

Bedtime Feeding (Example)

Bread . . . . .2 slices
Roast beef, lean . . . . . .2 oz.
Grapes 12
Mustard . . . . .as desired

2500 Calories (approximately)

carbohydrate . . . . . . .315 gm
protein . . . . .120 gm
fat . . . . .85 gm

Breakfast

2 Fruit Exchanges (List 3)
3 Bread Exchanges (List 4)

1 Meat Exchange (List 5)
2 Fat Exchanges (List 6)
1 cup nonfat milk (List 1)

Breakfast (Example)

Orange juice . . . . .1 cup
Cereal, dry . . . . .3/4 cup
Toast . . . . .2 slices
Egg 1
Margarine . . . . .2 tsp.
Nonfat milk . . . . .1 cup

Midmorning Feeding

1 Bread Exchange (List 4)
1/2 cup nonfat milk (List 1)

Midmorning Feeding (Example)

Graham crackers . . . . .2 squares
Nonfat milk . . . . .1/2 cup

Lunch

2 Meat Exchanges (List 5)

3 Bread Exchanges (List 4)
3 Fat Exchanges (List 6)

2 Vegetable Exchanges (List 2)
1 Fruit Exchange (List 3)
1 cup nonfat milk (List 1)

Lunch (Example)

Triple-decker sandwich:
    Cold cuts . . . . .1 1/2-oz.
                                          slice
    Cheese . . . . .1 oz.
    Bread . . . . .3 slices
    Mayonnaise-type
    dressing . . . . .2 tsp.
    Margarine . . . . .2 tsp.
Carrot and celery sticks 1 cup
Apple . . . . .1 small
Nonfat milk . . . . .1 cup

Midafternoon Feeding

1 Bread Exchange (List 4)
1 Fruit Exchange (List 3)

Midmorning Feeding (Example)

Saltine crackers 6
Pineapple juice . . . . . . .1/3 cup

Dinner

3 Meat Exchanges (List 5)
3 Bread Exchanges (List 4)

2 Vegetable Exchanges (List 2)
Vegetable(s) as desired (List 2)
1 Fruit Exchange (List 3)
3 Fat Exchanges (List 6)
1 cup nonfat milk (List 1)

Dinner (Example)

Chicken, baked   ......3 oz.
Peas ....1/2 cup
Potatoes, mashed ......1/2 cup
Bread ....1 slice
Tomatoes ....1 cup
Lettuce, radishes   .....as desired
Fruit cocktail   ....1/2 cup
Margarine ....3 tsp.
Nonfat milk ....1 cup

Bedtime Feeding

2 Bread Exchanges (List 4)
2 Meat Exchanges (List 5)
1 Fat Exchange (List 6)

1/2 cup nonfat milk (List 1)

Bedtime Feeding (Example)

Hamburger bun 1
Roast beef, lean   ......2 oz.
Mayonnaise-type
   dressing   ....2 tsp.
Nonfat milk ....1/2 cup

3000 Calories (approximately)

carbohydrate ....300 gm
protein ....140 gm
fat ....135 gm

Breakfast

1 Fruit Exchange (List 3)
3 Bread Exchanges (List 4)

2 Meat Exchanges (List 5)
4 Fat Exchanges (List 6)

1 cup 2% fat milk (List 1)

Breakfast (Example)

Orange juice ....1/2 cup
Cereal, dry ....3/4 cup
Toast ....2 slices
Eggs 2
Bacon crisp ....2 slices
Margarine ....2 tsp.
Milk, 2% fat ....1 cup

Midmorning Feeding

1 cup 2% fat milk (List 1)
1 Bread Exchange (List 4)

Midmorning Feeding (Example)

Milk, 2% fat ....1 cup
Graham crackers   .....2 squares

Lunch

3 Meat Exchanges (List 5)
3 Bread Exchanges (List 4)
3 Fat Exchanges (List 6)

1 Vegetable Exchange (List 2)
1 Fruit Exchange (List 3)
1 cup 2% fat milk (List 1)

Lunch (Example)

Sandwich:
  Cheese ....1 oz.
  Mayonnaise-type
  dressing ....2 tsp.
  Bread ....1 slice
Sandwich:
  Cold cuts ....two
           1 1/2-oz.
           slices

  Mayonnaise-type
  dressing ....2 tsp.
  Margarine ....1 tsp.
  Bread ....2 slices
Carrot and celery sticks 1/2 cup
Apple ....1 small
Milk, 2% fat ....1 cup

Midafternoon Feeding

1 Meat Exchange (List 5)
2 Bread Exchanges (List 4)

Midafternoon Feeding (Example)

Frankfurter 1
Frankfurter roll 1

Dinner

3 Meat Exchanges (List 5)
2 1/2 Bread Exchanges (List 4)

1 Vegetable Exchange (List 2)
Vegetable(s) as desired (List 2)
1 Fruit Exchange (List 3)
1 cup 2% fat milk (List 1)
3 Fat Exchanges (List 6)

Dinner (Example)

Chicken, baked ......3 oz.
Peas ....1/2 cup
Potatoes, mashed .....1/2 cup
Bread ....1/2 slice
Tomatoes ....1/2 cup
Lettuce, escarole .....as desired
Fruit cocktail ....1/2 cup
Milk, 2% fat ....1 cup
Margarine ....3 tsp.

Bedtime Feeding

1 Meat Exchange (List 5)
2 Bread Exchanges (List 4)
2 Fat Exchanges (List 6)
1 cup 2% fat milk (List 1)

Bedtime Feeding (Example)

Roast beef, lean ......1 oz.
Hamburger bun 1
Margarine ....2 tsp.
Milk, 2% fat ....1 cup
Mustard ....as desired

APPETIZERS AND BEVERAGES

One serving is equivalent to 3½ ounces or 100 grams.

When using basic ingredients such as arrowroot, eggs, flour, margarine, and tapioca, refer to Weights, Measures, and the Metric System, Notes on Special Ingredients Used in Recipes, and Additional Suggestions (see Contents).

HONOLULU DIP

Exchanges per serving: ¼ cup = 2 Fat
Calories per serving: 90 (for dip only)   Yield: 1½ cups

½ cup chopped fresh (or
   crushed, artificially
   sweetened) pineapple
2 tablespoons chopped mint

3 ounces Neufchâtel
   cream cheese
2 tablespoons safflower
   mayonnaise

Blend ingredients together. Serve with crisp carrot and celery sticks and crackers.

GOLDEN SHOYU DIP

Exchanges per serving: 2 tablespoons = 2 Fat
Calories per serving: 90   Yield: 1¼ cups

1 cup safflower mayonnaise
¼ cup soy sauce

½ teaspoon instant onion
¼ teaspoon arrowroot

Blend all ingredients until smooth. Chill. Restir before serving as dip for all fish "pupus," or with grilled or fried fish.

CHEESE NIBBLERS

Exchanges per serving: 1 ball = ¼ Bread, ⅔ Fat, ¼ Meat
Calories per serving: 60   Yield: 36 nibblers

½ cup sharp cheddar cheese,   ½ cup diet margarine
  grated   1 cup flour

Mix ingredients together and roll into balls. (These can be made ahead of time and frozen.) To bake, place in a preheated 375°F. oven for 15 minutes. If frozen, bake for 20–25 minutes.

CHEESE AND PINEAPPLE PUPUS

Exchanges per serving: ⅓ cup dip = 5 Fat, ½ Lean Meat
                       ½ cup pineapple = 1 Fruit
Calories per serving: 250   Yield: Fruit, 4 cups
                                        Sauce, 3 cups

1 whole fresh pineapple,   1 cup cheddar cheese,
  cubed*   grated
1½ cups diet mayonnaise   ½ cup shredded unsweet-
                                    ened coconut

Serve pineapple chunks on picks with other ingredients in bowls. Dip pineapple first in mayonnaise, then in cheese and coconut.

RUMAKI

Exchanges per serving: 4 Rumaki = 2 Fat, ½ Meat
Calories per serving: 125   Yield: 48 rumakis

12 chicken livers   1 cup water chestnuts,
1 teaspoon seasoned salt   drained
⅛ teaspoon ginger   16 slices bacon

Cut livers into small bite-sized pieces and season with salt and ginger; cut water chestnuts into halves and bacon into thirds. Wrap each piece

*1 average pineapple makes approximately 4 cups.

of liver with a half chestnut in bacon and secure with a pick. Broil or bake in 425°F oven until golden brown (25–30 minutes). Serve with hot fruit chutney, chili sauce, Chinese mustard, or Hot Shoyu Sauce (see Index).

YUMMY COFFEE DRINK

Exchanges per serving: 1 cup = 2 Fat
Calories per serving: 90   Yield: 4½ cups

2 cups strong iced coffee
Non-nutritive sweetener
   equivalent to ⅓ cup
   sugar

½ cup nondairy whipped
   topping
2 cups artificially sweetened
   ginger ale

Mix coffee and sweetener. Fill 4 large glasses about ¼ full with crushed ice. Whip nondairy topping. Add to each glass ¼ cup topping and ¼ cup coffee mixture, then ½ cup ginger ale. Stir slightly.

APPLE FOAM

Exchanges per serving: ⅓ cup = 1 Fruit
Calories per serving: 40   Yield: 2 cups

2 cups apple juice
1 teaspoon lemon juice
¼ cup egg whites
Dash of cinnamon

Non-nutritive granulated
   sweetener equivalent to
   1½ cups sugar (reserve
   ½ teaspoon)

Chill juices. Mix ½ teaspoon reserved sweetener with cinnamon, set aside. Beat egg whites until stiff; add balance of sweetener while beating. Add apple and lemon juice; pour into fruit cups. Sprinkle with the cinnamon-sweetener mixture.

COCOA

Exchanges per serving: 1 cup = 1 Nonfat Milk, ¼ Fat
Calories per serving: 90   Yield: 8 cups

6 tablespoons unsweetened
  cocoa
½ teaspoon salt
2 cups water

6 cups nonfat milk
Non-nutritive sweetener
  equivalent to ½ cup
  sugar

Mix cocoa, salt, and water. Stir constantly over very low heat for 2 minutes. Add milk and sweetener; continue stirring until cocoa comes to a boil. Serve.

HOT CHOCOLATE

Exchanges per serving: ½ cup = ½ Fat, ½ Nonfat Milk
Calories per serving: 75   Yield: 2½ cups

1½ ounces unsweetened
  chocolate
¾ cup water
Dash of salt

Non-nutritive sweetener
  equivalent to ½ cup
  sugar
2½ cups nonfat milk

Combine chocolate and water; cook, stirring constantly, until chocolate is melted. Add salt and sweetener; bring to boiling point; boil 4 minutes, stirring constantly. Place over boiling water, and gradually add milk, stirring constantly; heat. Just before serving, beat with rotary beater until frothy.

QUICK DRINK

Exchanges per serving: 1 cup = ½ Fruit, 1 Nonfat Milk
Calories per serving: 100   Yield: 1¼ cups

⅔ cup dry nonfat instant
  powdered milk
½ cup frozen fruit, un-
  sweetened, or ½ cup
  fresh fruit

Non-nutritive sweetener
  equivalent to 2 table-
  spoons sugar
2 ice cubes
2 tablespoons water

Blend all ingredients in blender until ice cubes are dissolved.

JOAN'S FRUIT SHAKE

Exchanges per serving: 1 cup = 1 Fruit, ½ Nonfat Milk
Calories per serving: 80   Yield: 4 cups

2 bananas
3 tablespoons fresh orange
  juice
Dash of salt

Non-nutritive sweetener
  equivalent to ½ cup
  sugar
⅛ teaspoon vanilla
2 cups nonfat milk

Blend ingredients until smooth and foamy. Place in refrigerator until chilled, then blend again. Serve.

CRANBERRY PUNCH

Exchanges per serving: ½ cup = 1 Fruit
Calories per serving: 40   Yield: 15 cups

8 cups artificially sweetened cranberry juice
  cocktail
3 cups unsweetened pine-
  apple juice

Non-nutritive sweetener
  equivalent to ½ cup
  sugar
4 cups artificially sweetened ginger ale

Combine juices and sweetener; chill. Stir in chilled ginger ale just before serving. Add ice cubes.

CRANBERRY SIP

Exchanges per serving: ½ cup = ¾ Fruit
Calories per serving: 30   Yield: 2½ cups

1 cup cranberries, washed
2 whole cloves
1 teaspoon cinnamon
1 cup water

Non-nutritive sweetener
  equivalent to 1½ cups
  sugar
¼ cup orange juice
¼ cup lemon juice
Dash of salt

Combine cranberries, spices, water, and sweetener; cook until cranberry skins burst. Strain; add remaining ingredients. Chill.

NONNIE'S CRANBERRY COCKTAIL

Exchanges per serving: ½ cup = 1 Fruit
Calories per serving: 40   Yield: 5 cups

4 cups artificially sweetened cranberry juice
3 cloves
1 stick cinnamon

Non-nutritive sweetener
  equivalent to 1 cup
  sugar
¼ cup fresh lemon juice
⅔ cup fresh orange juice
Dash of salt

Combine first four ingredients; bring to a boil. Reduce heat; simmer a few minutes, then remove from heat. Add citrus juices and salt; chill. Serve very cold.

APRICOT ORANGE PUNCH

Exchanges per serving: ½ cup = 1 Fruit
Calories per serving: 40   Yield: 7 cups

1½ cups artificially sweetened apricot nectar
3 cups fresh orange juice
½ cup fresh lemon juice

Non-nutritive sweetener
  equivalent to ½ cup
  sugar
2 cups artificially sweetened ginger ale

Combine first four ingredients; chill well. Just before placing in punch bowl, add well-chilled ginger ale.

COFFEE PUNCH

Exchanges per serving: 1 cup = 1 Nonfat Milk
Calories per serving: 80   Yield: 24 6-ounce cups

2 cups nonfat milk
8 cups strong coffee, cold
2 teaspoons vanilla
Non-nutritive sweetener
  equivalent to ½ cup
  sugar

4 cups ice milk (vanilla,
  chocolate, or coffee)
1 cup nondairy whipped
  topping
Dash of cinnamon or
  nutmeg

Combine milk, coffee, vanilla, and sweetener in large pitcher; stir until sweetener dissolves; chill. Place chunks of ice milk in punch bowl just before serving. Add coffee mix, top with nondairy whipped topping, stir lightly; sprinkle with cinnamon or nutmeg.

"DELISHUS" PUNCH

Exchanges per serving: ½ cup = 1 Fruit
Calories per serving: 40   Yield: 8 cups

1 dozen cloves, whole	1 cinnamon stick
1 orange, thinly sliced	1 teaspoon allspice
1 lemon, thinly sliced	2 tablespoons lemon juice
4 cups artificially sweet- ened cranberry juice cocktail	Non-nutritive sweetener to taste

Put a clove in each slice of orange and lemon. Place fruit slices in a pitcher. Combine cranberry cocktail and spices; heat to boiling over low heat. Add lemon juice; add sweetener to taste and strain hot mixture into pitcher over fruit. Serve in punch cups garnished with fruit slices.

OLGA'S MINTY DRINK

Exchanges per serving: 1 cup = ½ Fruit
Calories per serving: 22   Yield: 8 cups

¼ cup mint leaves, chopped fine	1 cup water
Non-nutritive sweetener equivalent to ½ cup sugar	½ cup fresh lemon juice 2 cups fresh orange juice 4 cups artificially sweet- ened ginger ale

Combine first three ingredients; bring to a boil. Cool and strain. When ready to serve, add remaining ingredients; pour over crushed ice in chilled glasses.

COLA DRINK

Exchanges per serving: 1 cup = 1 Nonfat Milk
Calories per serving: 80   Yield: 2 cups

2 teaspoons sugarfree,   Non-nutritive sweetener
  non-caloric cola   equivalent to 1 teaspoon
2 cups skim milk   sugar

Mix all ingredients well.

LEMONADE

Exchanges per serving: ½ cup = ½ Fruit
Calories per serving: 20   Yield: 2 cups

⅔ cup unsweetened lemon   Non-nutritive sweetener
  juice   to taste
1½ cups cold water   Lemon slices

Combine lemon juice and water. Sweeten with non-nutritive sweetener; add ice. Pour into large glasses over ice. Garnish with lemon slice.

LOU'S LEMONADE

Exchanges per serving: ½ cup = ½ Fruit
Calories per serving: 20   Yield: 8 cups

1 cup unsweetened lemon   6 cups water
  juice   1 cup artificially sweet-
Non-nutritive sweetener   ened cranberry juice
  equivalent to ¾ cup   cocktail
  sugar

Combine ingredients; mix well. Add ice cubes just prior to serving.

EGGNOG DIVINE

(Not for diabetics without consent of doctor.)
Exchanges per serving: ½ cup = ¼ Meat, ¾ Nonfat Milk
Calories per serving: 120   Yield: 5¼ cups
(alcohol is approximately 20)

3 eggs, separated
4 cups nonfat milk

Non-nutritive sweetener
    equivalent to ½ cup
    sugar
½ cup rum

Beat egg yolks until thick and lemony. Combine all ingredients except egg whites. Beat whites until stiff; fold in carefully just before serving.

NONALCOHOLIC EGGNOG

Exchanges per serving: 1 cup = ⅓ Skim Milk, ½ Meat
Calories per serving: 62   Yield: 4 cups

2 eggs
½ cup dry nonfat instant
    powdered milk
2⅔ cups water, ice cold

Non-nutritive sweetener
    equivalent to 2 table-
    spoons sugar
3 teaspoons vanilla
1 teaspoon rum flavoring

Place all ingredients in blender; mix well. Pour into cups and serve.

IMITATION WINE

Exchanges per serving: ½ cup = 1 Fruit
Calories per serving: 40   Yield: 8 cups

2 cups unsweetened grape
    juice
Non-nutritive sweetener
    equivalent to ½ cup
    sugar

2 cups artificially sweetened
    fruit-flavored carbon-
    ated beverage, chilled
4 cups artificially sweet-
    ened ginger ale, chilled

Combine juice and sweetener; chill. Stir in carbonated fruit-flavored beverage and ginger ale just before serving. Add ice cubes.

WINE LEMONADE

(Not for diabetics without consent of doctor.)
Exchanges per serving: 1 cup = none
Calories per serving: 168   Yield: 5½ cups
(alcohol is approximately 148)

3 cups water
½ cup fresh lemon juice

Non-nutritive sweetener
   equivalent to ½ cup
   sugar
2 cups white wine

Combine all ingredients; pour over crushed ice in chilled glasses.

SOUPS

JOAN'S JELLIED TOMATO CONSOMMÉ

Exchanges per serving: ⅔ cup = 1 Fat, ½ Fruit, 1 Vegetable
Calories per serving: 90   Yield: 3 cups

1 envelope unflavored
  gelatin
2¼ cups tomato juice
1 bouillon cube, any flavor
½ teaspoon salt
Non-nutritive sweetener
  equivalent to ¼ cup
  sugar
½ teaspoon Worcestershire
  sauce

⅛ teaspoon Tabasco sauce
2 tablespoons lemon juice
¼ cup cucumbers,
  unpeeled and diced
½ cup sour half-and-half or
  low-fat plain yogurt
  (optional)

Sprinkle gelatin over half the tomato juice in a saucepan. Add
bouillon cube; place over low heat, stirring constantly until gelatin
and cube are dissolved (about 3 minutes). Remove from heat. Add
rest of tomato juice, salt, sweetener, Worcestershire and Tabasco
sauces, lemon juice, and cucumbers. Pour into 2″ × 8″ × 8″ pan; chill
until firm. Spoon into serving dishes; serve with sour half-and-half or
plain lowfat yogurt, if desired.

ASPARAGUS SOUP

Exchanges per serving: ½ cup = 1 Vegetable
Calories per serving: 12   Yield: 5 cups

2 cups asparagus, cooked
3 cups water
4 bouillon cubes, any flavor

Dash of thyme
⅛ teaspoon salt
Dash of pepper

Purée asparagus. Boil water; combine with bouillon cubes, thyme,
salt, and pepper; add asparagus; simmer 5 minutes.

CUCUMBER SOUP

Exchanges per serving: 1 cup = 1 Vegetable
Calories per serving: 35   Yield: 4 cups

2 beef or chicken bouillon
   cubes
2 cups water
1½ cups cucumber, sliced
½ cup plain yogurt made
   from skim milk

¼ teaspoon lemon peel,
   dried
Dash of seasoned salt
Dash of pepper
Dash of thyme

Bring bouillon cubes, water, and cucumber slices to boil. Cover and simmer until cucumber is tender (about 10 minutes). Cool and place in refrigerator. When cold, blend; add yogurt, lemon peel, and seasonings. Blend until smooth. Serve cold.

VEGETABLE SOUP, COLD
(GAZPACHO)

Exchanges per serving: ½ cup = 1 Vegetable
Calories per serving: 30   Yield: 5 cups

1 cup tomatoes, peeled and
   finely chopped
½ cup green pepper, finely
   chopped (remove core)
½ cup celery, finely
   chopped
½ cup cucumber, peeled
   and finely chopped
¼ cup green onion, finely
   chopped
2 teaspoons parsley,
   snipped
1 teaspoon chives, snipped

1 small clove garlic, minced
   (put through garlic press)
3 tablespoons tarragon
   wine vinegar
1 teaspoon garlic salt
¼ teaspoon pepper
1 teaspoon Worcestershire
   sauce
2 cups tomato juice
Tabasco sauce to taste
   (approximately 2 tea-
   spoons)

Combine ingredients in either a glass or a stainless steel bowl. Put half the mixture through blender. When thoroughly blended, return to bowl; mix well. Cover bowl and place in refrigerator to chill at least 4 hours; serve in chilled cups. This may also be served in place of a salad.

GREAT CARROT or BEAN SOUP

Exchanges per serving: 1 cup = 1⅓ Vegetable
Calories per serving: 35   Yield: 3 cups

1 cup water	¼ teaspoon thyme
2 bouillon cubes, any flavor	Dash of salt
2 scant cups carrots (or green beans, if preferred)	Dash of pepper

Heat water with bouillon cubes in saucepan; stir occasionally. Add carrots; purée until smooth. Add thyme, salt, and pepper.

TARRAGON SOUP

Exchanges per serving: ⅔ cup = ½ Fat, 1 Vegetable
Calories per serving: 40   Yield: 2⅓ cups

2 tablespoons onion, chopped	½ teaspoon dried tarragon
2 tablespoons celery, chopped very fine	½ teaspoon salt
1 tablespoon diet margarine	⅛ teaspoon pepper
2 cups tomato juice	Dash of Tabasco sauce, if desired

Sauté onion and celery in margarine until onion is golden; add remaining ingredients. Bring to a boil. Lower heat; simmer 5 minutes.

EASY PEANUT SOUP

Exchanges per serving: ⅔ cup = 1 Bread, ½ Meat, ½ Fat
Calories per serving: 134   Yield: 4¾ cups

1½ cups cream of chicken soup	¼ cup chunky peanut butter
1½ cups cream of celery soup	1½ cups water

Blend all ingredients well; let simmer 5 minutes.

POTATO AND WATERCRESS SOUP

Exchanges per serving: 1 cup = ¾ Bread, ½ Nonfat Milk
Calories per serving: 111   Yield: 3⅓ cups

1⅓ cups cream of   ½ teaspoon thyme
  potato soup   Dash of salt
1⅓ cups nonfat milk   Dash of pepper
½ cup watercress, chopped
  fine (packed tightly)

Heat cream of potato soup with milk in saucepan. Purée watercress
and thyme. Mix with soup until well blended. Add salt and pepper.
Cook 4 or 5 minutes over medium heat (or until hot). Serve hot or
cold.

CELERY BEAN SOUP

Exchanges per serving: 1 cup = 1 Fat, ½ Nonfat Milk, ½ Vegetable
Calories per serving: 102   Yield: 4 cups

1 cup string beans, cut fine   Dash of salt
⅛ cup water   ⅔ teaspoon arrowroot
2 tablespoons onion,   powder
  chopped fine   1½ cups nonfat milk
1¼ cups cream of
  celery soup

Combine beans and onion with water, soup, and tiny dash of salt.
Cook in tightly covered saucepan about 6–7 minutes, until onions
soften. In another saucepan combine a few grains of salt and arrowroot powder; stir in milk gradually to make a smooth mixture. Add to
first mixture; cook over low heat, stirring occasionally until thickened. Adjust seasoning to taste.

FESTIVE TOMATO SOUP

Exchanges per serving: 1 scant cup = 1 Bread, 1 Fruit
Calories per serving: 140   Yield: 5⅔ cups

2⅔ cups condensed
   tomato soup

⅔ cup unsweetened
   orange juice concentrate
2½ cups water

Put tomato soup in pan; add mixture of orange juice and water. Boil gently. Serve hot or cold.

SHRIMP CHOWDER
(High cholesterol)

Exchanges per serving: 1 cup = 1 Bread, 2 Meat, ½ Nonfat Milk,
                        1 Vegetable
Calories per serving: 281   Yield: 7½ cups

½ cup onion, finely
   chopped
1 tablespoon diet margarine
2 cups water
2 teaspoons salt
1¼ cups potatoes, pared
   and cubed (about
   ½" thick)

2 cups nonfat milk, scalded
12 ounces shrimp, drained
   and shelled (if shrimp are
   large cut into smaller
   pieces)
½ tablespoon arrowroot
1 tablespoon water
Dash of salt
Dash of pepper

Sauté onion in margarine until golden. Add water, salt, and potatoes. Boil gently, covered, until potatoes are tender (about 20 minutes). Add scalded skim milk and shrimp, stirring occasionally. Bring to boil, reduce heat; simmer until shrimp are pink and cooked (about 5 minutes). Make smooth thin paste of arrowroot and water; add to chowder and stir until slightly thickened. Add pepper and remaining salt, to taste.

SPLIT PEA SOUP

Exchanges per serving: 1 cup = 1½ Bread, 1 Vegetable
Calories per serving: 132   Yield: 6 cups

1 cup green split peas
1 carrot, sliced thin
1 onion, sliced thin
5 cups water

3 beef or chicken bouillon
  cubes
1 teaspoon salt
Dash of pepper
1 teaspoon curry powder
  (optional)

Soak peas 2 to 3 hours in cold water; drain. Mix other ingredients except curry powder together in a saucepan. Cover and boil gently until peas are very soft (about 45 minutes). Stir in curry powder, if desired; press mixture through sieve and return purée to saucepan. Reheat and serve.

TURKEY-WATERCRESS SOUP

Exchanges per serving: 1 cup = 3 Lean Meat, 2 Vegetable
Calories per serving: 256   Yield: 3 cups

1 cup water
1⅓ cups condensed
  turkey broth
2 tablespoons onion,
  chopped fine
¼ cup celery, chopped fine
½ teaspoon salt

1½ cups cooked turkey, cut
  in small pieces
1 cup watercress, chopped
  fine (firmly packed)
1½ teaspoons arrowroot
2 tablespoons water

Simmer first six ingredients about 15 minutes. Add watercress and simmer again until watercress is wilted. Mix arrowroot and 2 tablespoons water into a smooth paste; stir into soup. Cook until clear and smooth (a few minutes).

QUICK AND TASTY CHICKEN SOUP

Exchanges per serving: 1 cup = 2¾ Lean Meat
Calories per serving: 185   Yield: 4 cups

1½ cups chicken, cooked
   and diced
1⅓ cups chicken broth
1 cup water
2 tablespoons onion,
   chopped fine

¼ cup celery, diced fine
½ teaspoon salt
½ teaspoon thyme
½ tablespoon arrowroot
1 tablespoon water

Simmer first seven ingredients for about 10 minutes. Make paste of arrowroot and 1 tablespoon water; add to soup. Cook until clear and smooth (takes just a few seconds).

SALADS

NOTES

We are listing below products that may be available to you:

Light 'n Lively Reduced Calorie Mayonnaise: 1 tablespoon = 40 calories

Kraft Catalina Low Calorie Dressing: 1 tablespoon = 25 calories

*Kraft Low Calorie Chunky Blue Cheese Dressing: 1 tablespoon = 16 calories

Kraft Low Calorie Creamy Cucumber Dressing: 1 tablespoon = 16 calories

*Kraft Low Calorie Chef Style Dressing: 1 tablespoon = 4 calories

Kraft Low Calorie French Style Dressing: 1 tablespoon = 21 calories

Kraft Low Calorie Italian Dressing: 1 tablespoon = 7 calories

Kraft Low Calorie Russian Dressing: 1 tablespoon = 30 calories

Kraft Low Calorie Thousand Island Dressing: 1 tablespoon = 50 calories

*Roka Brand Low Calorie Blue Cheese Dressing: 1 tablespoon = 13 calories

Wish-Bone Lite Dressing: 1 tablespoon = 13 calories

Regular mayonnaise: 2 tablespoons = 200 calories

Mayonnaise whip: 2 tablespoons = 138 calories

Regular French Dressing: 2 tablespoons = 150 calories

Diet French Dressing: 2 tablespoons = 42 calories

(Note: Calories can be reduced by 5 to 15 calories with Imitation Mayonnaise or 25 calories with Diet Salad Dressing.)

Vegetables that are so low in calories as to be unnecessary to count are celery, chicory, Chinese cabbage, endive, escarole, lettuce, parsley, peppers, radishes and watercress.

*Limited Distribution.

SWEET AND SOUR CUCUMBER SALAD

Exchanges per serving: ½ cup = 1 Vegetable
Calories per serving: 20   Yield: 2 cups

½ cup water
1 cup cider vinegar
Non-nutritive sweetener
   equivalent to 2 table-
   spoons sugar

2 tablespoons dill pickle,
   chopped fine
1½ teaspoons salt
2 cucumbers, sliced thin
1 stalk celery, sliced thin

Boil water, vinegar, sweetener, pickle, and salt. Place cucumbers and celery slices in glass jar; pour boiling liquid over; cover and refrigerate overnight. Drain before serving.

MARINATED VEGETABLE TOSS

Exchanges per serving: ½ cup = 1 Vegetable
Calories per serving: Yield: 8 ½-cup servings
   20 (excluding dressing)

2 cups fresh tomato wedges,
   peeled
½ cup radishes, sliced
½ medium red onion,
   thinly sliced

½ cup celery crescents
½ cup cucumber chunks
Dietetic Italian dressing

Combine all vegetables in salad bowl; pour Italian dressing over. Refrigerate overnight.

RADISH CELERY SALAD

Exchanges per serving: ½ cup = 1 Vegetable
Calories per serving: 8   Yield: 2 cups

1 cup radishes, sliced thin
1 cup celery, sliced thin

¼ cup French dressing
   (low-calorie)
1 cup lettuce leaves, torn up

Toss radishes, celery, and dressing together. Refrigerate an hour or so before placing on lettuce leaves.

SWEET AND SOUR BEETS

Exchanges per serving: 1 serving = ½ Med. Fat Meat, 1½ Vegetable
Calories per serving: 77   Yield: 6 servings

4 cups sliced beets
   (reserve juice)
Non-nutritive sweetener
   equivalent to 3 table-
   spoons sugar
1 teaspoon salt

¼ teaspoon black pepper
1 tablespoon allspice
½ cup vinegar
3 eggs, hard-boiled and
   shelled
2 cups lettuce, torn up

Mix ½ cup beet juice with sweetener, salt, pepper, and allspice. Boil gently about 5 minutes. Strain; stir in vinegar. Place eggs and beet slices in baking dish. Pour beet-juice mixture over; refrigerate overnight, turning both beets and eggs occasionally. Slice eggs with egg slicer; drain beets and divide into 6 servings. Place on lettuce leaves; top each with liquid; use half an egg for each serving.

CARROT SLICES

Exchanges per serving: ⅔ cup = ½ Bread, 1 Vegetable
Calories per serving: 54   Yield: 3 cups

2 cups carrots, scraped
   and cut into 1″ slices
¾ cup water
¼ cup cider vinegar
½ teaspoon dill pickle,
   chopped fine
1 tablespoon green onion
   seasoning

½ teaspoon poultry
   seasoning
½ teaspoon thyme
¼ teaspoon garlic salt
½ teaspoon marjoram
½ teaspoon seasoned salt
Dash of lemon pepper
1 cup prepared croutons

Simmer first nine ingredients, covered, until carrots are tender. Add salt, pepper, and croutons. Cool. Place in refrigerator for an hour, drain, and serve.

MOTHER'S RAW SPINACH SALAD

Exchanges per serving: 1 cup = 3½ Fat, 1 Vegetable
Calories per serving: 186   Yield: 5 servings

2 bunches fresh spinach
½ medium red onion, sliced
  thin and ringed
6 slices bacon, chopped
  and fried crisp

½ cup diet mayonnaise
½ cup wine vinegar
Non-nutritive sweetener
  equivalent to ½ cup
  sugar

Wash spinach thoroughly; cut off stems; crisp in refrigerator. Tear
into bite-size pieces into salad bowl; add onion rings and bacon bits.
Combine mayonnaise, vinegar, and sweetener; mix well in blender or
mixer. Pour over greens. Toss and serve at once.

HOT POTATO SALAD

Exchanges per serving: 1 cup = 1 Bread, 1 Lean Meat, 1 Vegetable
Calories per serving: 138   Yield: 4 cups

2 cups potatoes, pared
  and cubed
Water
2½ teaspoons salt
1 onion, chopped fine

1 stalk celery, chopped fine
¼ cup green pepper
  chopped fine
1 cup low-fat cottage cheese
2 cups lettuce leaves

Place potatoes in water to cover; cook until tender; drain. Toss potato
cubes and remaining ingredients together; mix well. Serve on lettuce
leaves.

TOMATO AND HERB SALAD

Exchanges per serving: 1 serving = 1 Vegetable
Calories per serving: 22   Yield: 6 servings

6 small tomatoes, peeled	4 tablespoons malt vinegar
1½ teaspoons oregano	½ teaspoon seasoned salt
Non-nutritive sweetener	¼ teaspoon pepper
equivalent to 1 table-	1 cup lettuce leaves, torn up
spoon sugar	

Chop 1½ tomatoes fine; combine with oregano, sweetener, vinegar, and salt. Slice remaining tomatoes, place on top of lettuce leaves; top with vinegar mix; refrigerate until ready to serve.

FROZEN ORANGE FRUIT SALAD

Exchanges per serving: ½ filled orange = 2 Fat, 1 Fruit
Calories per serving: 199   Yield: 8 servings
(+ approximately 10 per tablespoon whipped topping)

4 oranges	1 cup unsweetened fruit
¾ cup cream cheese*	cocktail, drained, or
½ cup diet mayonnaise or	mixed unsweetened fruits
diet salad dressing	¼ cup slivered almonds
1 tablespoon lemon juice	½ cup nondairy whipped
¼ teaspoon prepared	topping sweetened to
mustard	taste with artificial
¼ teaspoon salt	sweetener

Cut oranges in half and scoop out pulp. Combine cream cheese, mayonnaise, lemon juice, mustard, and salt. Add fruit cocktail, almonds, and drained orange pulp. Fold in whipped topping. Heap salad in orange halves; freeze until firm. Wrap individually in foil and keep frozen until needed. Remove from freezer ½ hour before serving. Garnish with endive or mint.

*See selections under Cheese and Egg recipes.

PEPPER SLAW

Exchanges per serving: 1 cup = 1 Vegetable
Calories per serving: 26   Yield: 3 cups

½ head cabbage
1 carrot, chopped fine
¼ green pepper, chopped
   fine

2 cups water
1 tablespoon mayonnaise-
   type dressing

Cut cabbage into small wedges. Place half in blender along with water, carrot and pepper. Blend quickly; turn off and drain at once, using liquid for blending with balance of cabbage, drain once more. Mix with mayonnaise dressing.

CAESAR SALAD

Exchanges per serving: 1 cup = 2 Fat, 1 Lean Meat, 1 Vegetable
Calories per serving: 150   Yield: 6 servings

1 clove garlic
2 cups romaine lettuce *or*
   2 cups iceberg lettuce
¼ cup olive oil
Juice of 1 lemon
¼ cup wine vinegar

2-ounce can anchovy fillets,
   drained and chopped
¼ cup Parmesan cheese
½ cup prepared croutons
1 egg, well beaten
Salt and pepper to taste

Rub salad bowl with cut clove of garlic. Tear cleaned and crisped lettuce into bite-size pieces in salad bowl. Pour olive oil, lemon juice, and vinegar over greens; toss lightly. Sprinkle chopped anchovies, grated cheese, and croutons on top; add beaten egg. Season. Toss and serve at once.

JELLIED FRUIT SALAD

Exchanges per serving: ⅔ cup = ¾ Fruit
Calories per serving: 31   Yield: 4 cups

1 envelope low-calorie
   strawberry gelatin
   dessert
1¾ cups boiling water
¼ cup fresh lemon juice

Non-nutritive sweetener
   equivalent to ½ cup
   sugar
1 cup fresh peaches, sliced
   fine
1 cup cantaloupe balls

Dissolve gelatin in boiling water. Add lemon juice and sweetener. Chill until consistency of thick syrup; add fruits. Place in lightly oiled mold and chill until set.

MOLDED BEET-ONION SALAD

Exchanges per serving: ½ cup = 1 Vegetable
Calories per serving: 25   Yield: 4 servings

1 envelope black raspberry
   diet gelatin
2 cups boiling water

1 cup shoestring beets,
   drained
5-ounce jar cocktail pickled
   onions

Dissolve gelatin in boiling water. Chill until consistency of egg whites. Fold in vegetables. Pour in pan or molds; refrigerate until firm (5–6 hours).

PEACH-Y SALAD

Exchanges per serving: ⅔ cup = 1½ Fruit
Calories per serving: 69   Yield: 4 cups

4 cups artificially sweetened peaches, halved
1 tablespoon vinegar

2 sticks cinnamon
½ teaspoon allspice
1 teaspoon cloves, whole
2 cups torn lettuce leaves

Mix peaches, vinegar, cinnamon, and allspice. Boil gently 5 minutes. Place in refrigerator 5–6 hours. Drain thoroughly; stick a clove in each peach half; serve on lettuce.

ANN'S APPLE SALAD

Exchanges per serving: ½ cup = ½ Lean Meat, 1 Fat, ½ Fruit
Calories per serving: 80   Yield: 4 servings

½ cup apples, thinly sliced
½ cup low-fat cottage
  cheese
2 tablespoons diet salad
  dressing

½ cup carrots, grated
½ cup celery, chopped fine
Dash of salt
1 cup torn lettuce leaves

Toss together first six ingredients. Divide mixture and place about ½ cup portions on lettuce. Refrigerate before serving.

SUPER SALAD

Exchanges per serving: ⅔ cup = 1 Fruit, ½ Vegetable
Calories per serving: 58   Yield: 5 servings

1 cup carrots, grated
2 cups unsweetened pine-
  apple tidbits (reserve
  syrup)
¼ teaspoon salt
½ teaspoon anise seed,
  crushed

1 tablespoon white vinegar
½ cup boiling water
⅛ cup lemon juice
1 envelope unflavored
  gelatin
2 cups torn lettuce leaves

Mix carrots, pineapple, salt, anise seed, vinegar, and water. Stir together lemon juice, gelatin, syrup from pineapple; let soften; add to first mixture. Pour into lightly oiled salad mold. Refrigerate until firm. Loosen mold in hot water; run table knife along inside edges, invert on lettuce.

JELLIED APPLESAUCE SALAD

Exchanges per serving: ½ cup = 1 Fruit
Calories per serving: 54   Yield: 4 servings

1 envelope diet raspberry
   gelatin
1¾ cups boiling water
1 cup unsweetened
   applesauce

½ cup unsweetened crushed
   pineapple, drained
½ cup celery, chopped

Dissolve gelatin in hot water. Let cool in refrigerator until the consistency of egg whites. Add fruits and celery; stir well. Pour into pan or molds and refrigerate until set (4–5 hours).

APPLE-CELERY-CRANBERRY-NUT MOLD

Exchanges per serving: ¾ cup = 1½ Fat, 1 Fruit
Calories per serving: 101   Yield: 4¼ cups

2 cups cranberries
1¼ cups water
Non-nutritive sweetener
   equivalent to 1 cup
   sugar
1 envelope unflavored
   gelatin

1 cup apples, peeled and
   diced
½ cup celery, chopped fine
½ cup pecans, chopped
   very fine
Lettuce

Cook cranberries in 1 cup water. When skins are broken, rub through sieve. Add sweetener and reheat. Soften gelatin in remaining ¼ cup water; add to cranberry purée; cool. When mixture starts to thicken, add apples, celery, and pecans. Pour into mold. Chill. Serve on lettuce.

GOLDEN GLOW SALAD

Exchanges per serving: ½ cup = ½ Fruit, ½ Vegetable
Calories per serving: 37   Yield: 4 cups

1 envelope unflavored
  gelatin
⅛ cup lemon juice
2 cups artificially sweetened pineapple tidbits
  (reserve juice)

¼ teaspoon salt
1 tablespoon vinegar
1 cup carrots, grated
½ cup boiling water
2 cups torn lettuce leaves

Mix gelatin, lemon juice, and juice from pineapple tidbits. Soften gelatin a few minutes; stir in salt, vinegar, carrots, pineapple, and boiling water. Pour into 9 × 5 × 3 loaf pan; refrigerate until firm (about 4 hours). Serve on lettuce bed.

RASPBERRY RHUBARB SALAD

Exchanges per serving: ½ cup = 1 Vegetable
Calories per serving: 20 (excluding dressing)   Yield: 4 cups

1 envelope dietetic rasp-
  berry gelatin
1 cup boiling water
½ cup artificially sweet-
  ened cooked rhubarb
½ teaspoon anise seed,
  crushed fine

½ cup apples, chopped fine
½ cup celery, chopped fine
1 or 2 drops red vegetable
  coloring
2 cups lettuce, chopped

Dissolve gelatin in water. Add rhubarb and anise seed; mix well. Cool until congealed slightly. Add apples and celery; mix well. Pour into slightly oiled 1 quart salad mold; chill until firm. Divide equally on lettuce and serve with fruit salad dressing, if desired.

MOLDED VEGETABLE SALAD

Exchanges per serving: ½ cup = ½ Vegetable
Calories per serving: 17   Yield: 4 servings

1 envelope diet orange
  gelatin
2 cups boiling water
½ cup white cabbage,
  chopped

½ cup carrots, shredded
¼ cup celery, finely
  chopped
¼ teaspoon celery seeds

Dissolve gelatin in boiling water. Chill until consistency of egg white. Fold in vegetables and celery seeds. Pour in 1 quart mold and refrigerate until firm.

CUCUMBER-PINEAPPLE-GELATIN SALAD

Exchanges per serving: ½ cup = ½ Fruit
Calories per serving: 23   Yield: 3½ cups

1 envelope diet lemon or
  orange gelatin
½ cup hot water
1 cup artificially sweet-
  ened dietetic pineapple
  tidbits with juice

¼ cup lemon or orange
  juice
⅛ teaspoon salt
1½ cups cucumber,
  shredded and drained

Dissolve gelatin in hot water. Drain pineapple, reserving ¼ cup juice. Add pineapple liquid, orange or lemon juice, and salt to gelatin. Chill until thickened and consistency of syrup. Fold in pineapple and cucumber. Pour into 1 quart mold and chill.

LAURA'S JELLIED VEGETABLE SALAD

Exchanges per serving: 1 serving = 1 Vegetable
Calories per serving: 23   Yield: 8 servings

2 envelopes unflavored
  gelatin
½ cup cold water
3 cups boiling water
½ cup fresh lemon juice
Non-nutritive sweetener
  equivalent to ⅔ cup
  sugar

1 tablespoon tarragon
  vinegar
1 teaspoon salt
3 drops food coloring
½ cucumber, diced fine
8 or 9 radishes, sliced
8 or 9 scallions, sliced

Soften gelatin in cold water; add boiling water; stir to dissolve. Blend
in lemon juice, sweetener, vinegar, salt, and coloring; chill until
mixture begins to thicken. Fold in vegetables and place in a lightly
oiled 1½ quart mold. Chill until set.

SEAFOOD SALAD

Exchanges per serving: ½ cup = 2 Fat, 2 Lean Meat
Calories per serving: 280   Yield: 4 servings

½ pound deveined shrimp,
  shelled, cooked, chilled,
  and cut in 2″ pieces
1 tablespoon green onion,
  minced
3 tablespoons diet salad
  dressing
3 tablespoons diet French
  dressing

½ cup chopped almonds
1 cup low-fat cottage cheese
2 cups lettuce, torn up
1 tomato, cut in wedges
1 teaspoon parsley sprigs,
  chopped fine

Mix first six ingredients. Divide evenly on lettuce; garnish with
tomato and parsley.

MEAT or SEAFOOD SALAD
(Suitable for salads or sandwich fillings)

Exchanges per serving: 3 tablespoons = 1 Fat, 1 Lean Meat
Calories per serving: 75   Yield: 3 cups

2 cups minced meat, shell-
fish, or flaked fish
1 tablespoon green onion,
minced
¼ cup celery, minced
1 teaspoon pimento,
minced
1 teaspoon fresh parsley,
minced, or parsley flakes

1 egg, hard-cooked,
chopped fine
1 teaspoon capers, minced
½ cup diet mayonnaise or
diet salad dressing
Salt and pepper to taste
Garlic salt to taste

Combine first seven ingredients. Mix with mayonnaise or salad dressing; season to taste. Chill.
Suggestions: Serve as sandwich filling with plain bread or toasted bun.
Serve as main-plate salad:

1. On bed of chopped lettuce, garnished with curled strips of carrot.
2. Stuffed in tomato or avocado.

EASY SALAD DRESSING

Exchanges per serving: 1 tablespoon = None
Calories per serving: 6   Yield: 1¼ cups

1 egg, well beaten
½ teaspoon salt
Dash of pepper
½ teaspoon dry mustard

½ cup vinegar
¼ cup skim milk
Non-nutritive sweetener
equivalent to ½ cup
sugar

Mix all ingredients except sweetener; cook until mixture comes to a racing boil, over low heat. Add sweetener; cool. Use for salads.

VINEGAR DRESSING

Exchanges per serving: None
Calories per serving: 0   Yield: ⅓ cup

¼ cup vinegar
2 tablespoons water
1 clove garlic, crushed
⅛ teaspoon salt
⅛ teaspoon paprika

Non-nutritive sweetener
  equivalent to 3½ tea-
  spoons sugar
½ teaspoon dill *or* tarragon,
  or a combination of
  rosemary and thyme

Combine all ingredients. Store in jar in refrigerator. Shake well before using.

NONFAT MILK DRESSING

Exchanges per serving: 1 tablespoon = None
Calories per serving: 4   Yield: 3 cups

1 cup white vinegar
Non-nutritive sweetener
  equivalent to ¾ cup
  sugar

2 cups nonfat milk

Beat all ingredients thoroughly with rotary beater. Store in refrigerator. May be used for lettuce, coleslaw, and so on.

SALLY'S SALAD DRESSING

Exchanges per serving: 1 tablespoon = None
Calories per serving: 2   Yield: 3 ounces or 5 tablespoons

2 teaspoons minced onion
4 tablespoons malt or
  cider vinegar

Non-nutritive sweetener
  equivalent to ½ cup
  sugar
2 teaspoons seasoned salt
½ teaspoon lemon pepper

Mix all ingredients well. Serve on fruit or vegetable salads or for coleslaw mix.

FRUIT SALAD DRESSING

Exchanges per serving: 1 tablespoon = None
Calories per serving: 3   Yield: ¾ cup

Non-nutritive sweetener
  equivalent to 3 cups
  sugar
½ cup unsweetened lemon
  juice
½ cup water

½ tablespoon arrowroot
½ teaspoon celery seed
½ teaspoon chervil
1 teaspoon celery salt
½ teaspoon dry mustard
½ teaspoon paprika

Combine sweetener, lemon juice, water, and arrowroot in a small pan; stir to blend. Add remaining ingredients and bring to a boil, cooking until thick and clear (about 3–4 minutes), stirring constantly. Cool; store in refrigerator.

LOW-CALORIE DRESSING

Exchanges per serving: 2 tablespoons = None
Calories per serving: 14   Yield: 1½ cups

1¼ cups condensed
  tomato soup
¼ teaspoon onion salt

⅛ teaspoon black pepper
¼ teaspoon garlic powder
3 tablespoons wine vinegar
1 tablespoon corn relish

Mix all ingredients together in large jar. Cover and refrigerate. Shake before using.

DRESSING À LA BLANCHE

Exchanges per serving: 1 tablespoon = None
Calories per serving: 4   Yield: 3 cups

1 cup white vinegar
2 cups skim milk

Non-nutritive sweetner
  equivalent to ¾ cup
  sugar

Place all ingredients in covered glass jar; shake until well mixed. Store in refrigerator. Use for lettuce, coleslaw, and so on.

MARGE'S SALAD DRESSING

Exchanges per serving: 1 tablespoon = None
Calories per serving: 7   Yield: 1½ cups

1 egg, well beaten
Non-nutritive sweetener
   equivalent to ⅔ cup
   sugar
⅔ cup nonfat milk

½ cup malt vinegar
1 teaspoon mustard
½ teaspoon salt
⅛ teaspoon pepper
½ teaspoon diet margarine

Combine all ingredients in top of double boiler and cook over hot water. Stir until thick and smooth. Chill. Use for vegetable salads.

GOURMET SOUR CREAM DRESSING

Exchanges per serving: 1 tablespoon = ½ Fat
Calories per serving: 25   Yield: 1¼ cups

2 tablespoons green onion,
   minced
3 tablespoons wine vinegar
Non-nutritive sweetener
   equivalent to 2 table-
   spoons sugar

1 teaspoon prepared mustard
⅛ teaspoon pepper
Dash of Tabasco sauce
1 cup low-calorie sour
   cream (calories = 17 per
   tablespoon with sour
   half-and-half)

Combine all ingredients. Chill at least 30 minutes to blend flavors.

GINNY'S SALAD DRESSING

Exchanges per serving: 1 tablespoon = None
Calories per serving: 0   Yield: 5 tablespoons

2 teaspoons onion juice
4 tablespoons cider vinegar
Non-nutritive sweetener
   equivalent to ½ cup
   sugar

⅛ teaspoon dry mustard
⅛ teaspoon pepper
⅛ teaspoon salt

Mix all ingredients well. Serve on fruit or vegetable salads or for coleslaw mix.

FRUIT DRESSING

Exchanges per serving: 1 tablespoon = ½ Fat
Calories per serving: 21   Yield: 3 cups

¼ teaspoon dry mustard
¼ teaspoon salt
1 teaspoon onion juice
1 cup cider vinegar
4 teaspoons paprika

4 tablespoons celery seed
1½ cups water
½ cup oil
Non-nutritive sweetener
    equivalent to 3 cups
    sugar

Combine first five ingredients. Bring to boil; simmer over low heat about 5 minutes; remove from heat. Add remaining ingredients. Chill. Serve on fruit salads.

LOUISE'S SALAD DRESSING

Exchanges per serving: 1 tablespoon = ½ Fat
Calories per serving: 17   Yield: 1 cup

3 egg yolks, beaten well
2 tablespoons nonfat milk
Non-nutritive sweetener
    equivalent to ½ cup
    sugar

½ cup fresh lemon juice
2 teaspoons diet margarine,
    melted
⅛ teaspoon salt

Mix all ingredients in saucepan; cook over medium heat, stirring constantly, until mixture comes to a boil and is slightly thick. Chill.

BLUE CHEESE TOPPING

Exchanges per serving: 1 tablespoon = None
Calories per serving: 9   Yield: 2¼ cups

2 cups plain low-fat
    yogurt

3 tablespoons low-calorie
    blue cheese dressing
½ teaspoon salt

Combine ingredients; chill. Serve on lettuce leaves, or baked potato.

SALAD DRESSING

Exchanges per serving: 1 tablespoon = None
Calories per serving: 8   Yield: 2 cups

2 eggs, well beaten
1 teaspoon salt
⅛ teaspoon lemon pepper
1 teaspoon dry mustard

1 cup malt or cider vinegar
1 cup nonfat milk
Non-nutritive sweetener
    equivalent to 1 cup
    sugar

Mix first six ingredients. Cook until mixture comes to a racing boil, over low heat. Add sweetener; cool.

CHUTNEY or CURRY MAYONNAISE

Exchanges per serving: 1½ teaspoons = 1 Fat
Calories per serving: 48   Yield: 1 cup

1 cup safflower mayonnaise
1 teaspoon any minced fruit

1 teaspoon chutney *or*
    curry powder

Blend all ingredients together for spicy sauce for seafoods and chicken salad.

FRENCH-STYLE VINEGAR DRESSING

Exchanges per serving: 1 tablespoon = 1½ Fat
Calories per serving: 65   Yield: ¾ cup

2 tablespoons vinegar
½ teaspoon salt
1 teaspoon paprika
4 tablespoons lemon juice

½ onion, grated fine
6 tablespoons oil
Non-nutritive sweetener
    equivalent to 1 cup
    sugar

Bring vinegar, salt, paprika, lemon juice, and onion to a boil. Cool. Add oil and sweetener; cook again until thick as desired.

THOUSAND ISLAND DRESSING

Exchanges per serving: 1 tablespoon = None
Calories per serving: 9   Yield: 1⅓ cups

1 cup unflavored low-fat
   yogurt
¼ cup catsup (See Index
   for recipe)
2 tablespoons celery,
   diced fine
1 tablespoon green pepper
   diced fine

1 tablespoon onion,
   chopped fine
Non-nutritive sweetener
   equivalent to ½ cup
   sugar
¼ teaspoon seasoned salt
¼ teaspoon pepper

Mix all ingredients; blend well. Chill overnight in refrigerator.

LUAU MAYONNAISE

Exchanges per serving: 1 tablespoon = 2 Fat
Calories per serving: 80   Yield: 1¼ cups

1 cup safflower mayonnaise
2 tablespoons artificially
   sweetened pineapple
   juice

1 tablespoon maraschino
   cherry syrup

Thin mayonnaise with juice and syrup; blend to smooth pink color.

DOTTIE'S FRENCH DRESSING

Exchanges per serving: 1 tablespoon = 2 Fat
Calories per serving: 90   Yield: ¾ cup

½ cup olive oil
¼ cup malt vinegar
¼ teaspoon dry mustard

1 teaspoon salt
Dash of paprika
Dash of lemon pepper

Place all ingredients in glass jar. Blend or shake until well mixed.
Chill.

CHEESE AND EGG DISHES

NOTES

Cheeses, for the most part, are high in fat content since they are made from whole milk, often with cream added. See Meat Exchange List for categorized cheese choices. *Example:* Cheddar is a high-fat meat, whereas part-skim milk mozzarella is a medium-fat meat.

In the recipes, all Meat Exchanges are listed as "lean" with necessary added Fat Exchange accounted for.

Wherever possible bread and cereal products should be whole grain. Fiber is an important component in the diet. Recent research indicates that including fiber in the diet assists in the control of blood sugar.

The following cheeses are available in some areas; check your market:

Soft Diet Parkay Imitation Margarine: 1 tablespoon = 50 calories
Neufchâtel Cream Cheese: 3 tablespoons = 23 calories
*Golden Image Mild Imitation Cheddar Cheese: 1 ounce = 57 calories
*Golden Image Imitation Colby Cheese: 1 ounce = 55 calories
*Philadelphia Brand Imitation Cream Cheese: 1 ounce = 52 calories
Tasty Brand Imitation Pasteurized Processed Cheese Spread: 1 ounce = 75 calories
*Golden Image Imitation Pasteurized Processed Cheese Spread: 1 ounce = 48 calories
*Golden Image Imitation Pasteurized Processed Food Singles: 1¾-ounce slice = 38 calories

You may also find:

Kraft Low Calorie Imitation Grape Jelly: 1 tablespoon = 12 calories
Kraft Low Calorie Imitation Strawberry Preserves: 1 tablespoon = 14 calories

*Indicates limited distribution.

Fried eggs and omelets can be cooked beautifully in a Teflon-coated pan without the addition of fat.

When using basic ingredients such as arrowroot, eggs, flour, margarine, and tapioca, refer to Weights, Measures, and the Metric System, Notes on Special Ingredients Used in Recipes, and Additional Suggestions (see Contents).

FLUFF OMELET

Exchanges per serving: 1 serving = 1 Lean Meat, ½ Fat
Calories per serving: 73   Yield: 1 serving

1 egg   Dash of salt
1 tablespoon water

Using a wire whisk, beat all ingredients together. Place in Teflon pan and cook until done.
VARIATIONS: Diet Jelly: No additional calories.
Cheese: ½ ounce grated cheese, add 35 calories to above.
Ham and Green Pepper: 1 tablespoon ham and 1½ tablespoons chopped green pepper, add 35 calories to above.

EGGS CURRY

Exchanges per serving: 1 serving = 1 Bread, 2½ Lean Meat,
                                  ½ Nonfat Milk, 1 Vegetable
Calories per serving: 320   Yield: 4 servings

6 eggs, hard-boiled   1½ tablespoons arrowroot
¼ cup almonds, slivered   1 teaspoon salt
2 tablespoons diet   1½ teaspoons curry powder
   margarine   2 cups nonfat milk
1 onion, chopped fine   4 slices toast
½ cup celery, chopped fine

Thinly slice shelled eggs. Brown almonds in margarine until golden brown. Remove; drain on absorbent paper. In same pan sauté onion and celery until golden; stir in arrowroot, salt, and curry powder; stir in milk slowly. Cook, stirring constantly, until thick and smooth. Stir in sliced egg; heat to boil. Place a slice of toast in the bottom of each of four individual, heated casseroles. Divide eggs evenly over the toast; sprinkle with almonds.

SCRAMBLED EGGS

Exchanges per serving: 1 serving = 1 Lean Meat, ½ Fat
Calories per serving: 78   Yield: 1 serving

1 egg	salt
1 tablespoon nonfat milk	pepper

To eliminate the use of fat, scramble eggs in double boiler (or use Teflon-coated pan). Mix egg and milk with wire whip or fork; add salt and pepper and for variety, a dash of curry powder or chopped chives, green onion, or parsley. For a marvelous variation, add 2 tablespoons Spanish sauce to raw egg mixture, then cook.

OMELET WITH COTTAGE CHEESE

Exchanges per serving: 1 serving = 2 Fat, 3 Lean Meat
Calories per serving: 240   Yield: 2 servings

2 tablespoons diet margarine	½ cup low-fat cottage cheese, sieved
4 eggs, separated	Dash of pepper
Dash of salt	1 tablespoon chervil

Preheat oven to 350°F. Melt margarine in skillet. Beat egg whites with salt until stiff but not dry. Beat yolks separately until lemon-colored and thick; add cheese and pepper and beat until smooth. Fold in egg whites and chervil. Place mixture in skillet; cook over medium heat until lightly browned on bottom and fluffy (about 3–4 minutes). Place in oven 15 minutes; make a crease down center with knife and fold over. Serve at once.

EGGS ON TOAST, OVEN STYLE

Exchanges per serving: 1 serving = 1 Bread, 1 Fat, 1 Lean Meat
Calories per serving: 157   Yield: 6 servings

 6 slices bread   1 tablespoon chervil
 6 teaspoons diet   ⅛ teaspoon salt
   margarine   ⅛ teaspoon pepper
 6 eggs, separated

Preheat oven to 350°F. Butter each slice of bread with margarine; place buttered-side-up on cookie sheet. Beat egg whites until stiff; distribute evenly on bread slices. Make a hollow in center of each; fill with yolk. Sprinkle eggs with chervil, salt, and pepper. Bake until yolk is nearly set and white is lightly browned (about 15 minutes). Serve at once.

EGGS WITH CHEESE SAUCE

Exchanges per serving: 1 egg with ¼ cup sauce and 1 slice of toast =
                       1 Bread, 1½ Lean Meat, 1 Fat
Calories per serving: 183   Yield: 6 servings, 4 cups sauce*

 1¼ tablespoons arrowroot   ½ cup nonfat milk
 ½ teaspoon salt   1 tablespoon diet
 Dash of cayenne   margarine
 1 tablespoon prepared   1½ cups (5 ounces) cheddar
   mustard   cheese, grated
 1 tablespoon chervil   6 eggs
                               6 slices bread

Preheat oven to 350°F. Butter individual custard cups. Mix first five ingredients together; stir in milk slowly. Continue stirring over medium heat until thick and smooth. Remove from heat; stir in margarine and cheese. Stir until cheese has melted and sauce is smooth. Break one egg into each cup; cover with ¼ cup cheese sauce. Bake until firm (15–20 minutes). Toast bread; cut in half; serve egg with toast.

*Refrigerate balance of sauce for use another time.

CHEESE TOAST AND EGGS

Exchanges per serving: 1 serving = 1 Bread, 2 Lean Meat, 1 Fat
Calories per serving: 230   Yield: 4 servings

4 slices bread   4 eggs, poached
4 ounces mozzarella cheese

Preheat oven to 350°F. Toast bread; top each slice with 1 oz. cheese.
Put on cookie sheet; place in oven until cheese just melts (2–3
minutes). Add poached egg on top. Serve at once.

SALLY'S CHEESE FONDUE

(Not for diabetics without consent of doctor.)
Exchanges per serving: 1 slice = 1 Bread, ⅔ Meat
Calories per serving: 168   Yield: 12 servings

1 clove garlic, peeled   Dash of pepper
2 cups dry white wine   Dash of salt
2 cups cheese, shredded   Dash of nutmeg
    fine*   12 slices firm bread, cut
¼ teaspoon arrowroot   into cubes, leaving one
2 tablespoons Kirschwasser   side of crust on each cube
    (if approved by doctor)

Rub an earthenware casserole with garlic, then add wine. Heat slowly
over chafing dish burner. Mix cheese lightly with arrowroot; when
bubbles in wine rise to surface, add cheese mix a handful at a time.
Stir each handful until it melts; continue until all cheese is melted.
Add Kirschwasser and seasonings; stir well. Turn heat low but keep
fondue slowly bubbling. Have each person take a cube of bread on the
end of a fork and twirl it in the bubbling fondue. If fondue is too thick,
add a little *hot* wine.

*This could be Swiss cheese made with skim milk.

HAM AND CHEESE ON BUNS

Exchanges per serving: ½ bun = 1 Bread, 2 Lean Meat
Calories per serving: 193   Yield: 6 servings

3 hamburger buns, sliced across
6 1-ounce slices baked ham
¼ cup dietetic cranberry sauce

6 1-ounce slices skim-milk mozzarella cheese or 6 ounces cheese grated, divided into 6 servings

Toast bun halves slightly; top each with slice of ham. Spread each with cranberry sauce; place thin slice of cheese (or 1 ounce grated) over this; put under broiler until cheese melts and is lightly browned.

BLINTZES WITH CHEESE FILLING

Exchanges per serving: 1 blintz = ¾ Bread, 1 Lean Meat
Calories per serving: 100   Yield: 1 dozen

1 cup flour
½ teaspoon salt
½ teaspoon baking powder
1 cup nonfat milk
3 eggs
2 tablespoons diet margarine, melted

2 cups low-fat cottage cheese, sieved
Non-nutritive sweetener equivalent to 2 tablespoons sugar
½ teaspoon cinnamon
¼ teaspoon allspice or nutmeg

Sift flour, salt, and baking powder together. Beat milk, 2 eggs, and margarine. Slowly add to flour mixture; stir to form thin batter. Grease frying pan lightly, then pour ⅛ cup (2 tablespoons) batter into skillet; tilt skillet to cover bottom completely. Cook until top of pancake is firm; turn onto paper towel, with uncooked side down on waxed paper. Make rest of pancakes, greasing skillet as necessary. Mix cottage cheese, sweetener, cinnamon, allspice or nutmeg, and remaining egg. Top each pancake, with tablespoon of filling. Fold over sides, then the ends, to make small drugstore-type package; set to one side. Refrigerate until ready to serve. A few minutes before serving, melt margarine in skillet and lightly brown each blintz, starting with flap side down. Turn and brown on other side. Serve warm.

FISH, MEAT, AND POULTRY

NOTE: All meat recipes are given as lean meat portions with necessary fat allowances noted, to avoid confusion regarding lean-, medium-, and high-fat categories of meat.

CHOP SUEY WITH TUNA

Exchanges per serving: 1 cup = 1 Bread, 1 Lean Meat
Calories per serving: 130   Yield: 4 servings

2 stalks celery, cut small
½ onion, chopped fine
2 cups + 2 tablespoons water
¾ cup rice
Non-nutritive sweetener equivalent to ½ teaspoon sugar

Dash of pepper
2 tablespoons soy sauce
¾ cup water-packed tuna, drained (or any cooked poultry could be substituted for a different dish)

Cook celery and onion in 2 tablespoons water over low heat, covered. When tender, remove from heat; add rice, 2 cups water, and seasonings; bring to boil. Turn heat low and cook, covered, until rice is tender and liquid absorbed (about 30 minutes). Add tuna. Mix and remove from heat; set aside, covered, for a few minutes before serving.

NOTE: If desired, you can add ⅔ cup of canned, fresh or frozen chop suey vegetables for more nutrition. This would add 35 calories per serving.

CHEESE AND CRAB ORIENTAL STYLE

Exchanges per serving: 1 serving = ¼ Bread, 2½ Lean Meat,
2 Vegetable, 1 Fat
Calories per serving: 225   Yield: 5 servings

½ cup mushrooms, sliced
½ carrot, sliced thin
¼ cup green pepper, diced
1 cup celery, sliced
1 cup onion, chopped fine
2 tablespoons oil
Non-nutritive sweetener
  equivalent to 1 table-
  spoon sugar

1 teaspoon salt
1 bay leaf
4 cups tomatoes, fresh or
  canned
¾ cup rice, precooked
1½ cups crab meat, frozen,
  thawed, and drained
½ cup sharp cheese, grated

Preheat oven to 350°F. Sauté first five ingredients in oil in Dutch
oven or other ovenproof container until onion is golden brown. Add
sweetener, salt, bay leaf, and tomatoes; boil for 5 minutes, gently.
Stir in rice and crab meat. Sprinkle entire mixture with grated cheese.
Bake 20–25 minutes.

FISH AND MUSHROOMS

Exchanges per serving: 1 serving = 1 Fat, 3 Lean Meat, 1 Vegetable
Calories per serving: 200   Yield: 4 servings

1 onion, sliced thin
1 tablespoon oil
1½ cups mushrooms, sliced
  thin
1 pound fish fillets (cod,
  halibut, sole) cut in
  1″ slices

Dash of salt
Dash of pepper
1 stalk celery, sliced thin
1 tablespoon soy sauce
1 tablespoon dry sherry

Preheat skillet and sauté onion in oil. Add mushrooms and sauté
about 2 minutes, stirring constantly, until mushrooms wilt. Spread
half of fillet slices on mushrooms; sprinkle with salt and pepper; add
remaining fillets; sprinkle these with salt and pepper. Add celery, soy
sauce, and sherry; cook gently, covered, for ten minutes.

HARRIET'S FISH DISH

Exchanges per serving: 1 serving = ½ Fat, 3 Lean Meat, 2 Vegetable
Calories per serving: 220   Yield: 4 servings

2 onions, sliced thin
1 clove garlic, crushed
1 tablespoon diet
  margarine
½ cup parsley, snipped
½ teaspoon salt
⅛ teaspoon pepper

2 cups canned tomatoes
1 tablespoon tomato paste
2 chicken bouillon cubes
4 4-ounce fish fillets or
  steaks, about ¾" thick
3 slices tomato, cut thin
3 slices lemon, cut thin

Preheat oven to 300°F. Sauté onions and garlic in margarine until golden; add parsley, salt, pepper, tomatoes with juice, tomato paste, and bouillon cubes. Simmer gently, uncovered, about 20 minutes. Place fish steaks in medium baking dish. Cover with sauce; top with tomato slices and lemons. Bake until tender.

BAKED FISH STEAKS

Exchanges per serving: 3 ounces = Fat, 3 Lean Meat, ¼ Vegetable
Calories per serving: 236   Yield: 4 servings

4 3-ounce fish steaks (halibut, swordfish, or
  similar)
3 teaspoons oil
1 onion, sliced thin

1 potato, sliced thin
½ carrot, sliced thin
Dash of salt
Dash of pepper
½ teaspoon parsley,
  snipped

Preheat oven to 450°F. Remove skin from fish steaks; cut meat away from bone. Cut four 10" × 12" pieces of heavy duty foil, use oil to grease center of each piece of foil; place a steak on each piece of foil. Top each steak with slices of onion, potato, and carrot, and salt and pepper. Using drugstore folds, wrap each piece separately. Put on cookie sheet and bake until fish flakes and is tender, approximately 20 minutes. Garnish with parsley.

HILO FILLET OF SOLE

Exchanges per serving: 3 ounces = 2 Fat, 3 Lean Meat
Calories per serving: 256   Yield: 8 servings

1½ pounds fish fillets (cod, halibut, sole)
¼ teaspoon salt
2 teaspoons instant minced onion
1½ teaspoons water
¾ cup safflower mayonnaise

1 teaspoon lemon juice
¼ teaspoon seasoned salt
1 teaspoon parsley, finely chopped
⅓ cup chopped macadamia nuts, or slivered almonds

Wipe fillets with damp cloth; sprinkle with salt. Roll and secure each with toothpick. Place rolls in steamer or on wire rack above boiling water; cover and steam 15 minutes. Mix onion, water, mayonnaise, lemon juice, seasoned salt, and parsely. Remove fillets carefully from steamer; spread quickly with mayonnaise mixture. Top with nuts and serve at once.

SHRIMP AND RICE

Exchanges per serving: ½ cup rice and ¾ cup sauce = 1 Bread, 3 Lean Meat, 1 Vegetable
Calories per serving: 227   Yield: 4 servings

2 cups tomatoes
2 tablespoons parsley flakes
2 cups celery, sliced thin
¼ teaspoon basil
1½ teaspoons salt
⅛ teaspoon pepper

½ teaspoon oregano
3-ounce can tomato paste
2 7-ounce packages frozen, deveined, shelled shrimp
½ cup long-grain rice

Mix everything except rice and shrimp in large skillet, stirring occasionally. Boil gently, uncovered until celery is nearly tender (about 30 minutes). Stir in shrimp; boil until shrimp are cooked but still tender (about 5–10 minutes). Cook rice as directed, omitting margarine or butter. Serve shrimp over rice.

CRAB, SHRIMP, RICE SUPREME
(Moderate cholesterol)

Exchanges per serving: ¾ cup = ½ Bread, 3 Fat, 1½ Lean Meat
Calories per serving: 228   Yield: 10 servings

2 cups cooked rice
1 cup diet mayonnaise
½ cup green onion, chopped
¼ cup green pepper, chopped
1 cup tomato juice

¼ cup toasted almonds, slivered
8 ounces fresh, frozen, or canned crab meat
8 ounces fresh, frozen, or canned shrimp
¼ cup prepared bread crumbs

Preheat oven to 350°F. Mix all ingredients except bread crumbs together; place in casserole and top with bread crumbs. Bake 1 hour. Use fresh seafood if available. This is an excellent party casserole as it can be made a day ahead and refrigerated.

TUNA (or SALMON) PIE WITH CRUST

Exchanges per serving: 1 serving = 1 Bread, ½ Fat, 3 Lean Meat
Calories per serving: 258   Yield: 6 servings

1 cup long-grain white rice, uncooked
2 tablespoons diet margarine
3 eggs
1¼ cups water-packed tuna (or pink salmon), drained and flaked

¼ teaspoon salt
⅛ teaspoon pepper
⅛ teaspoon nutmeg
¾ cup American cheese, grated
¾ cup nonfat milk, scalded
½ teaspoon parsley

Preheat oven to 400°F. Cook rice as directed; mix with margarine and one egg. Line a 9″ pie pan; mound rice mixture up to about 1″ above rim of plate. Spread tuna (or salmon) in shell; sprinkle with salt, pepper, nutmeg, and cheese. Beat remaining eggs in small bowl; stir in scalded milk. Return to pan and heat until smooth; pour mixture over cheese. Bake until cheese is dark golden brown (about 30 minutes). Sprinkle parsley over top.

SALMON (or TUNA) CASSEROLE

Exchanges per serving: ½ cup = ¼ Bread, ½ Fat, ¼ Nonfat Milk,
1½ Lean Meat
Calories per serving: 130   Yield: 24 ½-cup servings

1 cup dry noodles,
  uncooked
2 cups mushrooms, sliced
  thin
4 tablespoons onion,
  chopped fine
4 tablespoons diet
  margarine
1 teaspoon salt

¼ teaspoon pepper
½ cup flour
2 teaspoons paprika
2 cups nonfat milk
2 cups half-and-half
4 cups pink salmon (or tuna,
  water-packed and well
  drained)
1 cup Parmesan cheese,
  grated

Preheat oven to 375°F. Cook noodles according to directions on the
package. Sauté mushrooms and onion in margarine until tender; stir
in salt, pepper, flour, and paprika. Stir in milk slowly, cooking and
stirring constantly until thick and smooth. Remove from heat; stir in
half and half. Remove skin and bones from drained salmon (or
tuna), then flake. Mix fish with noodles, mushroom mixture, and all
but a little of the grated cheese. Pour into casserole; sprinkle remaining cheese on top. Bake 20–25 minutes.

SWEET-SOUR TONGUE

Exchanges per serving: 1 oz. = 1 Meat, ¼ Fat
Calories per serving: 105   Yield: 3 servings

2 tablespoons diet
  margarine
1 tablespoon arrowroot
½ teaspoon salt
Non-nutritive sweetener
  equivalent to 2 table-
  spoons sugar

2 tablespoons malt vinegar
¼ teaspoon pepper
1 cup stock
3 ounces cooked smoked
  tongue, sliced

Blend first six ingredients with stock; cook until thickened. Add
tongue and heat.

STUFFED BUNS

Exchanges per serving: 1 bun = 1½ Bread, 1½ Fat, 1 Lean Meat
Calories per serving: 232   Yield: 8 servings

6-ounce can diet water-
  packed tuna (or chicken
  or turkey)
2 tablespoons green onion,
  minced
2 tablespoons celery,
  minced
1 tablespoon ripe olives,
  chopped

Minced dill pickle to taste
½ cup diet mayonnaise
¼ cup cheddar cheese,
  grated
8 frankfurter buns

Mix first seven ingredients; fill buns with mixture. Wrap in foil.
Place in 350°F. oven about 10–15 minutes until hot and cheese has
melted.

ONION, LIVER, AND CHEESE
(High cholesterol)

Exchanges per serving: 2 ounces liver = 1 Fat, 2 Lean Meat
                       1 tablespoon cheddar cheese = ½ Fat
Calories per serving: 168   Yield: 6 servings

1 pound beef liver,
  quartered
1 tablespoon flour
Dash of salt
Dash of pepper

Dash of garlic salt
2 tablespoons diet
  margarine
½ cup cheddar cheese,
  grated
1 onion, sliced very thin

Remove skin and veins from beef liver; cut into ½" serving pieces.
Sprinkle lightly with flour; shake off excess and sprinkle salt, pepper,
and garlic salt on each side. Sauté liver in margarine a few mintues
over medium heat. Turn off heat. Pour off most of margarine; return
pan to burner; sprinkle pieces with cheese, then thin rounds of onion.
Cover; heat until cheese is melted. Serve.

LIVER À LA BOURGEOISE
(High cholesterol)

Exchanges per serving: 3½ to 4 oz. = ½ Fat, 3–4 Lean Meat,
½ Vegetable

Calories per serving: 120   Yield: 8 servings

1 carrot, shredded
1 onion, minced
1 turnip, diced
1 bay leaf
2 tablespoons diet
  margarine

1 tablespoon arrowroot
2½ pounds beef liver*
2 cups water
Dash of seasoned salt
Dash of lemon pepper

Brown carrot, onion, and turnip with the bay leaf in margarine. Add arrowroot and blend. Add liver and water. Season and simmer 1½ to 1¾ hours.

FRANKFURTER CASSEROLE

Exchanges per serving: 1 serving = 1 Bread, 2 Fat, 1 Meat,
1 Vegetable

Calories per serving: 260   Yield: 8 servings

1¼ cup condensed bean and
  bacon soup
1¼ cups water
2 all-beef frankfurters (or
  chicken or turkey
  franks), cut into
  ½″ pieces

1 onion, chopped fine
1 green pepper, chopped
  fine
½ cup celery, chopped fine
2 tablespoons prepared
  mustard
1 cup ready-mix biscuit
  mixture, prepared as
  package directs

Preheat oven to 375°F. Mix all ingredients except biscuits. Boil gently 5 minutes. Put 6 slices into each of 8 individual baking dishes; add about ¾ cup mixture; top each with biscuit. Bake until biscuits are dark golden brown (about 20 minutes). Serve at once.

*Note: 5 oz. with shrinkage = 3½ to 4 oz. servings.

CALIFORNIA POT ROAST

Exchanges per serving: 2 ounces meat = 2 Lean Meat
Calories per serving: 125   Yield: 20 servings

4 pounds beef rump roast	2 carrots, sliced
2 tablespoons flour	1 tablespoon Worcester-
1 teaspoon salt	shire sauce
Dash of pepper	1 cup water
1 tablespoon oil	Non-nutritive sweetener
1 onion, chopped fine	equivalent to ½ cup
	sugar

Dredge meat well in flour, salt, and pepper. Brown in oil in skillet; add remaining ingredients. Cover; simmer about 4 hours over low heat.

ROAST BEEF WITH FRUIT SAUCE

Exchanges per serving: 1 ounce = 1 Lean Meat
                       ¼ cup sauce = 1 Fruit
Calories per serving: 43 (sauce)   Yield: 3 cups sauce
                      55 (meat)

3- to 4-pound rump/clod/	Salt and pepper to taste
round/sirloin-cut roast	
(lean meat group)	

Trim fat from beef before roasting. Salt and pepper. Place roast on rack; bake at 325°F for 1½ hours. Trim remaining fat after roasting.

SAUCE

4 cups artificially sweet-	⅓ cup unsweetened frozen
ened plums (reserve	orange juice concentrate
syrup)	2 tablespoons Worcester-
¼ teaspoon salt	shire sauce
⅛ teaspoon pepper	⅛ teaspoon Tabasco sauce
1 tablespoon arrowroot	

Drain and pit plums. Save ¾ cup syrup. Purée plums until smooth; add syrup and remaining ingredients. Blend until smooth. In medium saucepan, heat to boiling. Serve over Roast Beef.

HAMBURGER CORNMEAL SHEPHERD'S PIE

Exchanges per serving: 1 serving = 1 Bread, 3 Fat, 2 Lean Meat,
　　　　　　　　　　　　　　　1 Vegetable
Calories per serving: 322　　　　　　　　　　　Yield: 8 servings

½ cup green pepper, chopped fine	1 teaspoon chili powder
¼ cup onion, minced fine	½ cup flour, sifted
16 ounces (1 lb.) lean ground round (15% fat)	¾ cup yellow cornmeal
5 tablespoons oil	Non-nutritive sweetener equivalent to 1 tablespoon sugar
1 cup tomato sauce	2 teaspoons baking powder
2 tablespoons low-calorie catsup (See Index)	½ teaspoon thyme
2 teaspoons salt	1 egg
Dash lemon pepper	½ cup nonfat milk

Preheat oven to 400°F. Sauté green pepper, onion, beef in 2 tablespoons oil in skillet, until beef is well browned. Stir in tomato sauce, catsup, 1 teaspoon salt, lemon pepper, and chili powder. Put into 1½ quart casserole. Stir flour, cornmeal, sweetener, baking powder, remaining salt, and thyme together in a bowl; add egg, milk, and remaining oil. Stir until smooth. Top the first mixture with the second; bake uncovered, until cornbread is slightly brown and firm to touch (about 30 minutes). Loosen cornbread with a knife around edges; turn onto serving plate with top side down.

MEAT CASSEROLE

Exchanges per serving: 4-ounce serving = 1 Bread, 3 Meat,
                            1 Vegetable

Calories per serving: 290   Yield: 4 servings
(will vary with meat used)

¾ cup noodles, uncooked
2½ cups tomato juice
2 cups celery, chopped fine
½ cup green pepper,
  chopped fine

2 cups lean beef, cut in 1"
  cubes, cooked
⅛ teaspoon pepper
1½ teaspoons salt
½ teaspoon diet margarine

Heat oven to 350°F. Combine all ingredients; turn into well-greased
casserole; bake 45 minutes.

SPAGHETTI AND SAUCE

Exchanges per serving: 1 serving = 1 Bread, 3 Lean Meat, 2 Fat,
                            1 Vegetable

Calories per serving: 292   Yield: 8 servings sauce;
                              ½ cup cooked spaghetti per serving

3 cups (1½ pounds) lean
  ground beef (15% fat)
1 cup onion, chopped fine
½ cup celery, chopped fine
2 cloves garlic, minced
  very fine
½ cup fresh mushrooms,
  sliced thin

2 tablespoons oil
¾ cup tomato paste
1½ cups tomato juice
2 teaspoons salt
Dash of pepper
2 ounces thin spaghetti
  per serving

Brown meat well; sauté onion, celery, garlic, and mushrooms in oil
until onion is golden brown. Add tomato paste, tomato juice, salt,
and pepper; cover; boil gently for 1½ hours. After cooling, refrigerate overnight. About 20 minutes before serving, cook spaghetti
according to package instructions; drain thoroughly. Measure sauce
and add enough water to make a total of 5 cups of sauce. Return sauce

to pan, cover and boil gently about 10 minutes. Place ½ cup cooked spaghetti on each plate; top with ⅔ cup meat sauce.

CHILI CON CARNE

Exchanges per serving: 1 serving = 1 Bread, 2 Meat, 1 Vegetable
Calories per serving: 170   Yield: 8 servings

1 pound coarse ground beef
  chuck (chili grind)
1 cup onion, chopped fine
1 clove garlic, crushed fine
2 tablespoons chili powder

1¼ cups condensed tomato
  soup
2 cups kidney beans
1 tablespoon malt vinegar
¼ teaspoon salt

Brown beef in hot skillet; drain in sieve and pat dry with paper towel; stir in onion, garlic, and chili powder. Cook, stirring often, until onion is tender. Add remaining ingredients; bring to boil. Reduce heat and simmer, uncovered, stirring occasionally, about 15 minutes.

POLLY'S CHILI CON CARNE

Exchanges per serving: 1 serving = 1 Bread, ½ Fat, 2½ Lean Meat,
                          1 Vegetable
Calories per serving: 283   Yield: 5 servings

1 cup onion, chopped fine
½ cup green pepper,
  chopped fine
2 cups celery, chopped fine
1 clove garlic, sliced thin
1 tablespoon oil

2 cups coarse ground chuck
  roast (no added fat)
2 cups kidney beans,
  thoroughly drained
2 cups tomatoes
1 tablespoon chili powder
½ teaspoon salt

Sauté onion, pepper, celery, and garlic in oil until onion is golden brown. Add beef; cook until well browned. Stir in kidney beans, tomatoes, chili powder, and salt; simmer uncovered about 45–50 minutes. Just before serving, taste to see if more chili powder is needed.

CORNED BEEF DINNER

Exchanges per serving: 3-ounce slice = 1 Bread, 2 Vegetables,
3 Lean Meat
Calories per serving: 300   Yield: 16 3-ounce servings

4-pound corned-beef
  round*
Water
6 onions
6 carrots

6 parsnips, scraped
3 potatoes (4 ounces each)
  peeled and scraped
6 cups cabbage

Cover meat with cold water in Dutch oven; bring to a boil; drain. Add water to cover; again bring to boil; reduce heat to low. Cover. Cook until meat is nearly tender (about 3 hours), skimming off as much fat as possible from cooking water. (If you remove meat from broth and refrigerate—or put in freezer, if time is short—fat will harden and remove easily.) Add vegetables; cook until vegetables are done (about 10–15 minutes more). Remove vegetables from water; drain and trim fat from meat.

STUFFED FLANK STEAK

Exchanges per serving: 2 ounces = ¼ Bread, ½ Fat, 2 Lean Meat
Calories per serving: 152   Yield: 16 servings

2-pound flank steak
Dash of salt
Dash of lemon pepper
1 tablespoon flour
4 cups bread cubes
2 small onions,
  chopped fine

¾ cup celery, chopped fine
1½ teaspoons sage
½ teaspoon Mei Yen
  seasoning
3 tablespoons diet
  margarine
½ cup water

Preheat oven to 350°F. Score steak lightly, crosswise. Sprinkle with salt and lemon pepper; dredge in flour; pound coating well into the steak. Combine next five ingredients; spread over steak. Roll meat and tie, or fasten edge with toothpicks. Brown in margarine, then add

*Brisket may be used but must account for 1 Fat Exchange per ounce of meat.

water; cover and cook about 1½ hours, until tender. Baste occasionally.

MEAT LOAF

Exchanges per serving: 1 serving = ½ Bread, 3 Lean Meat, 1½ Fat
Calories per serving: 258   Yield: 6 servings

1 egg
2 cups lean ground round
   (15% fat)
3 slices bread, cubed fine
¼ cup catsup (See Index)
⅓ cup onion, chopped fine

2 tablespoons green pepper,
   chopped fine
1 teaspoon salt
½ teaspoon dry mustard
1 tablespoon prepared
   horseradish, if desired

Preheat oven to 400°F. Mix all ingredients well. Form into a loaf. Place in foil-lined 5 × 9 pan; bake until done (15–20 minutes).

MEATBALLS WITH CARAWAY SEEDS

Exchanges per serving: 2 meatballs = ¼ Bread, 2 Lean Meat, 1 Fat
Calories per serving: 182   Yield: 8 servings

2 cups lean ground round
   (15% fat)
1 onion, minced fine
1 egg
1 teaspoon lemon peel,
   grated fine
¼ teaspoon pepper
½ teaspoon salt

1 tablespoon dried
   parsley flakes
8 ounces raw potato,
   coarsely grated
2½ cups water
4 beef bouillon cubes
1 teaspoon arrowroot
½ teaspoon caraway seeds
1 tablespoon water

Mix first eight ingredients; form into sixteen meatballs. Bring water to boil; dissolve bouillon cubes in water. Add meatballs; cover tightly. Gently boil about 30 minutes. Remove meatballs from broth; stir arrowroot and caraway seeds into 1 tablespoon water; stir into broth until thick and smooth. Pour a little gravy over meatballs; garnish with parsley, if desired. (Store remaining gravy in tightly covered jar in refrigerator for later use.)

MEATBALLS

Exchanges per serving: 2 meatballs = ½ Bread, 1 Lean Meat, ¼
Nonfat Milk, ½ Fat

Calories per serving: 135   Yield: 6 servings

2 cups lean ground round
  (15% fat)
¼ cup prepared
  bread crumbs
1 teaspoon salt
1½ cups buttermilk

¾ cup instant rice
1 teaspoon diet
  margarine
1 cup water
½ tablespoon arrowroot

Mix beef, crumbs, salt, ½ cup buttermilk, and rice. Shape into two
dozen meatballs (about 1″ round). In large skillet, brown meatballs in
margarine on all sides; pour water over; cover tightly. Boil until rice
is tender and meat is cooked (about 30 minutes). Remove from
skillet. Mix remaining 1 cup buttermilk with arrowroot to form
smooth paste; stir into liquid remaining in skillet. Stirring constantly,
cook until gravy is thick (do not boil). Return meatballs to pan and
gently heat. Serve with gravy.

ROAST LEG OF LAMB

Exchanges per serving: 3 ounces = 3 Lean Meat
Calories per serving: 156   Yield: 10–12 servings

5- to 6-pound leg
  of lamb
1 clove garlic
2–3 teaspoons Bouquet
  Garni

1 teaspoon ginger
1 teaspoon seasoned salt
1 teaspoon lemon pepper
2 tablespoons flour

Preheat oven to 300°F. Wipe meat with damp cloth. Do not remove
the fell (the paperlike covering over the meat). Make gashes in roast
with sharp knife; cut garlic into slivers and insert a piece in each gash.
Rub meat with seasonings; dredge with flour. Place, fat side up, in
shallow roaster. Roast uncovered until tender (about 30–35 minutes
per pound). Remove garlic and serve.

VEAL À LA KING

Exchanges per serving: 1½ ounces = ¼ Bread, 2 Lean Meat
Calories per serving: 346   Yield: 16 servings
                              (3 tablespoons each serving)

½ cup green pepper,
  chopped fine
½ cup mushrooms
3 tablespoons diet
  margarine
3 tablespoons arrowroot

4 cups nonfat milk
Dash of seasoned salt
Dash of pepper
4 cups cooked veal, diced
1 pimiento, diced
8 slices toast

Cook pepper and mushrooms in margarine for 8 minutes; remove vegetables. Add arrowroot to margarine; blend. Add milk and seasonings; cook until thickened, stirring constantly. Add green pepper, mushrooms, veal, and pimiento; heat. Spoon 3 tablespoons over each one-half slice toast.

SAUERKRAUT AND SPARERIBS

Exchanges per serving: 2 ounces meat and ½ cup sauerkraut =
                       2 Lean Meat, ½ Vegetable, 2 Fat
Calories per serving: 220   Yield: 6 servings

3 cups sauerkraut
Non-nutritive sweetener
  equivalent to ¼ cup
  brown sugar

4 pounds spareribs*
Dash of seasoned salt
Dash of pepper
½ cup hot water

Preheat oven to 350°F. Place sauerkraut in greased baking dish. Sprinkle with sweetener. Brown parboiled spareribs under broiler. Season, place on sauerkraut; add hot water. Cover. Bake 45 minutes to 1 hour.

*Approximately 8 ounces including bone, for 2 ounces meat. Parboil ribs to defat as much as possible.

HAM LOAF

Exchanges per serving: 1 serving = ½ Bread, 2 Lean Meat, 1 Fat
Calories per serving: 183   Yield: 16 servings

1½ pounds lean ham,
    ground well
1 pound lean ground beef
2 eggs, beaten
1¼ cups nonfat milk
4 slices soft bread, broken
    into small pieces
1½ teaspoons salt

Dash pepper
Non-nutritive sweetener
    equivalent to ¾ cup
    sugar
¼ teaspoon cinnamon
¼ teaspoon cloves
¼ teaspoon nutmeg
½ teaspoon dry mustard
½ teaspoon vegetable oil

Preheat oven to 350°F. Combine all ingredients except oil; mix well.
Use oil to grease loaf pan. Place mixture in pan. Bake 1½ hours.

BAKED HAM or HAM STEAK WITH PINEAPPLE

Exchanges per serving: 3 ounces = 1 Fruit, 3 Lean Meat
Calories per serving: 220   Yield: 24 servings

6-pound canned ham
Non-nutritive sweetener
    equivalent to ½ cup
    sugar
1 teaspoon dry mustard

½ cup bread crumbs
¾ cup pineapple juice
5–6 slices unsweetened
    pineapple

Preheat oven to 300°F. Place ham in baking dish. Spread ham with
mixture of sweetener, mustard, and bread crumbs. Add pineapple
juice. Bake 15 minutes. Add slices of pineapple and cook entire dish
an additional 45 minutes.

PORK ROAST WITH SPICE SAUCE

Exchanges per serving: 3 ounces = 3 Lean Meat
Calories per serving: 200   Yield: 12 servings

4-pound fresh pork picnic
  shoulder
Dash of salt
Dash of pepper
2 small onions, minced
1 tablespoon Worcester-
  shire sauce

Non-nutritive sweetener
  equivalent to 1½ cups
  sugar
½ teaspoon paprika
½ cup vinegar
½ cup water
2 tablespoons catsup
  (See Index)

Have butcher bone and roll roast. Salt and pepper roast; place fat side
up on rack in open roaster. Roast at 350°F. 40–45 minutes per pound.
Combine other ingredients; cook together for 5 minutes. Pour over
roast and serve.

PORK PATTIES IN GRAVY

Exchanges per serving: 1 serving = ½ Bread, 1 Fat, 2 Lean Meat,
                        1 Vegetable
Calories per serving: 225   Yield: 8 servings

2 cups very lean pork
  shoulder, trimmed of all
  visible fat, then ground
2 eggs
½ cup nonfat milk
4 slices dry bread, cubed
  fine
1 onion, chopped fine
1½ teaspoons salt

⅓ teaspoon pepper
¾ teaspoon nutmeg
2 tablespoons salad oil
½ cup water
8 onions, peeled
1¼ cups condensed beef
  bouillon
1 teaspoon oregano
¼ teaspoon paprika

Mix first eight ingredients well; let stand a few minutes. Divide
mixture into patties; brown well in oil on both sides. Drain on brown
paper or paper towel. Pour fat from pan; add remaining ingredients.
Return patties to mixture; cover and cook gently 30 minutes.

MAINE SUPPER

Exchanges per serving: 1 serving = 2 Bread, 1 Fat, 3 Lean Meat
Calories per serving: 325   Yield: 6 servings

1 tablespoon onion, chopped	Non-nutritive sweetener equivalent to 1½ cups brown sugar
2 tablespoons green pepper, chopped	
2 tablespoons diet margarine	½ cup celery, chopped
4 cups pork and beans	1 cup Vienna sausages, each sliced in half

Brown onion and pepper in margarine. Add pork and beans, sweetener, and celery. Mix together and divide among 6 individual casseroles. Place ¹⁄₆ of sausage pieces in each casserole; bake at 350°F. until browned.

CHARLOTTE'S CURRIED CHICKEN

Exchanges per serving: ½ cup sauce with chicken over ½ cup rice =
                    1 Bread, ½ Fruit, 2½ Lean Meat, 1 Vegetable
Calories per serving: 256   Yield: 6 servings

1 cup long-grain white rice	1 chicken bouillon cube
2 chicken breasts (16 to 18 ounces total) split, boned, and cut into 2″ to 3″ pieces	1 teaspoon salt
	1½ teaspoons curry powder
	½ tablespoon arrowroot
	¾ cup nonfat milk
1 tablespoon diet margarine	1 cup water
1 cup mushrooms, sliced thin	1 cup apples, sliced
½ cup onions, chopped fine	1 teaspoon parsley, chopped fine

Cook rice as directed, adding ½ tablespoon margarine. Sauté chicken, mushrooms, and onions in remaining ½ tablespoon margarine until chicken is lightly browned on all sides (about 15 minutes). Combine bouillon cube, which has been finely crushed, salt, curry powder, and some of the milk to make a smooth paste; then add remaining milk, water, apple, and parsley. Cook until thick and smooth and apple is tender, stirring constantly. Stir chicken into sauce; serve over the rice.

CHICKEN LIVERS

Exchanges per serving: 1 serving = 1 Fat, 3 Lean Meat, 1 Vegetable
Calories per serving: 231   Yield: 4 servings

2 onions, sliced thin
2 stalks celery, sliced thin
1 tablespoon diet margarine

1 pound chicken livers
½ teaspoon salt
¼ teaspoon pepper

Sauté onions and celery in margarine until celery is wilted. Remove vegetables, leaving fat in pan. Add chicken livers; turn heat high; cook, turning once or twice, until done (3–5 minutes). Top with onions and celery. Season with salt and pepper.

CHICKEN SUPERB

Exchanges per serving: 1 serving = 1 Fat, ¼ Fruit, 3 Lean Meat,
                          ¼ Bread
Calories per serving: 279   Yield: 4 servings

¼ cup flour
1 teaspoon salt
⅛ teaspoon pepper
2 chicken breasts, split
   and skinned
2 tablespoons diet
   margarine
½ green pepper, chopped
   fine

¼ cup pimiento, diced fine
½ cup mushrooms, cut
   in quarters
¼ teaspoon ginger
1 cup canned chicken
   broth
¼ cup orange juice
½ orange, unpeeled and
   sliced thin

Mix together flour, salt, half the pepper. Lightly coat chicken with flour mixture. Cook chicken in margarine until golden, using a tightly covered pan. Turn breasts meat side down; add remaining ingredients; cover. Stirring occasionally, simmer gently until tender (about 30 minutes).

BROILED SPRING CHICKEN

Exchanges per serving: 2 ounces = 2 Lean Meat
Calories per serving: 20   Yield: 8 2-ounce servings

2- to 3-pound broiling   Dash of seasoned salt
  chicken, dressed, cut   Dash of lemon pepper
  into serving pieces
2 tablespoons diet
  margarine, melted

Preheat oven to 500°F. Brush chicken with margarine; rub with salt
and pepper. Place under broiler; brown evenly; turn and brown other
side. Allow 30 minutes or more to cook so the joints are not rare.
Baste with pan juices from time to time, adding water if needed.

SAUCES

BERRY SAUCE

Exchanges per serving: 1 tablespoon = None;
$\frac{1}{4}$ cup = $\frac{1}{2}$ Fruit
Calories per serving: 5 (per tablespoon)   Yield: 1½ cups

Non-nutritive sweetener
   equivalent to ½ cup
   sugar
1 teaspoon arrowroot
Dash of salt
½ cup water

1 cup berries (for example,
   blueberries, raspberries)
1 tablespoon lemon juice
1 teaspoon lemon rind,
   grated

Combine sweetener, arrowroot, and salt; stir in water. Add berries. Bring to a boil; simmer until clear and thick, about 5 minutes. Remove from heat; add lemon juice and rind. Chill and use over ice creams, custards, plain cakes, waffles, or pancakes.

BARB'S BARBECUE SAUCE

Exchanges per serving: ½ cup = 2 Vegetable
Calories per serving: 45   Yield: 2 cups

½ cup onions, chopped fine
⅔ cup tomato paste
1 cup water
1 teaspoon Worcestershire
   sauce
2 teaspoons maple extract
2 tablespoons garlic-
   flavored vinegar

¼ cup catsup (see fol-
   lowing recipe)
1 teaspoon salt
⅛ teaspoon pepper
¼ teaspoon dried oregano,
   crushed fine
¼ teaspoon dried rosemary,
   crushed fine

Blend all ingredients together in a saucepan; simmer over low heat about 30 minutes, or until onions are well cooked. Use with any broiled meat such as lamb patties, ground beef, beef, pork, or lamb chops.

CATSUP

Exchanges per serving: 1 tablespoon = None
Calories per serving: 6   Yield: 2 cups

4 tomatoes, quartered
⅓ cup green pepper,
   chopped fine
2 tablespoons milk red
   pepper, chopped very
   fine
½ cup malt vinegar
½ teaspoon salt
Non-nutritive sweetener
   equivalent to 1 cup sugar

¼ teaspoon cinnamon
⅛ teaspoon allspice
⅛ teaspoon anise seed,
   crushed fine
¼ teaspoon ground mustard
¼ teaspoon powdered red
   pepper
¼ teaspoon mace

If using blender, fill ¾ full with first four ingredients; blend about
3–4 seconds at highest speed. If not using blender, mix until puréed.
Pour mixture into pan; add vinegar, salt, and sweetener. Tie spices
loosely together in a bag of cheesecloth and add. Simmer, uncovered,
until reduced by about half. Remove bag of spices.

GRAVY

Exchanges per serving: 1 tablespoon = None
Calories per serving: 4   Yield: 2 cups

1 onion, thinly sliced
2 stalks celery, diced
1¼ cups chicken broth (or
   condensed beef
   consommé)

1¼ cups water
¼ teaspoon Gravy Master
1 tablespoon arrowroot

Combine onion, celery, broth, and water in a medium saucepan;
cover and boil gently over low heat until onion is transparent. Strain.
Reserve vegetables for later use. Return broth to pan. Use a little
water, Gravy Master, and arrowroot to make a smooth paste; stir
slowly into borth and heat to boiling.

MINT SAUCE

Exchanges per serving: 1 tablespoon = None
Calories per serving: 0   Yield: 1¾ cups

¼ cup vinegar
1 cup water
½ cup mint leaves,
    chopped
¼ cup lemon juice

Non-nutritive sweetener
    equivalent to 1½ table-
    spoons sugar
½ teaspoon salt

Heat vinegar and ½ cup water to boiling. Pour over half the mint leaves. Let stand 15 minutes. Strain; add remaining water, lemon juice, sweetener, and salt; chill. Add remaining mint leaves just before serving. Serve with lamb.

SWEET AND TANGY TOMATO SAUCE FOR SPARERIBS AND LOIN OF PORK

Exchanges per serving: ½ cup = 1 Vegetable
Calories per serving: 28   Yield: 2½ cups

⅓ cup vinegar
Non-nutritive sweetener
    equivalent to 1½ cups
    sugar
2 tablespoons Worcester-
    shire sauce

2 tablespoons prepared
    mustard
½ teaspoon Tabasco sauce
¼ cup onion, minced
2 cups tomato sauce

Combine all ingredients in a saucepan; bring to a boil. Use to baste spareribs or loin of pork.

HOT SHOYU (SOY) SAUCE

Exchanges per serving: 2 tablespoons = None
Calories per serving: 8   Yield: 1⅔ cups

1 cup soy sauce
⅔ cup water
Non-nutritive sweetener
    equivalent to ½ cup
    brown sugar

¼ teaspoon instant onion
1 teaspoon arrowroot
    powder

Blend all ingredients; heat to light boil. Serve as dip for Shrimp Tempura or "pupus," or as sauce for fish or chicken.

BARBECUE SAUCE

Exchanges per serving: 1 tablespoon = None
Calories per serving: 2   Yield: 2 cups

4 tablespoons lemon juice
Dash of red pepper
2 tablespoons cider vinegar
1 cup low-calorie catsup
½ cup water (see
    catsup recipe)
3 tablespoons Worcester-
    shire sauce

Dash of lemon pepper
1½ teaspoons mustard
Non-nutritive sweetener
    equivalent to ½ cup
    sugar
½ teaspoon salt

Combine all ingredients; simmer over medium heat about 20–25 minutes.

COLD SHOYU (SOY) SAUCE

Exchanges per serving: 1 tablespoon = None
Calories per serving: 9   Yield: ¾ cup

½ cup soy sauce
Non-nutritive sweetener
    equivalent to 3 table-
    spoons brown sugar

2 tablespoons wine
    vinegar

Blend ingredients well. Serve in small bowls with hot fried foods, cold meat, or fish "pupus."

TOMATO SAUCE

Exchanges per serving: ¼ cup = 1 Vegetable
Calories per serving: 25   Yield: 3 cups

½ onion, chopped fine
1 tablespoon olive oil
½ clove garlic, minced fine
2 cups tomato sauce
1 cup water

¼ teaspoon basil
Non-nutritive sweetener
  equivalent to ¼ tea-
  spoon sugar
¼ teaspoon salt

Sauté onion in oil until lightly browned; add garlic and sauté until lightly browned. Stir in remaining ingredients; simmer 1 hour. If using for spaghetti, simmer 5 hours.

GOLDEN SHOYU DIP

Exchanges per serving: 1 tablespoon = 1½ Fat
Calories per serving: 78   Yield: 1¼ cups

1 cup safflower mayonnaise
¼ cup soy sauce

½ teaspoon instant onion
¼ teaspoon arrowroot

Blend all ingredients until smooth; cook until consistency desired; chill. Restir before serving as dip for all fish "pupus" or with grilled or fried fish.

SWEET AND SOUR MARINADE
For Shish Kabobs and Brochettes

Exchanges per serving: ½ cup = ½ Fruit
Calories per serving: 28   Yield: 2 cups

1 cup soy sauce
½ cup vinegar
½ cup unsweetened pine-
  apple juice

Non-nutritive sweetener
  equivalent to 1½ cups
  sugar
½ teaspoon salt
½ teaspoon garlic powder

Combine all ingredients; bring to a boil. Marinate beef or lamb cubes in mixture for at least four hours in the refrigerator. Also useful for basting meat while cooking.

TANGY TONGUE SAUCE

Exchanges per serving: ¼ cup = ½ Fat, ½ Fruit
Calories per serving: 56   Yield: 3¼ cups

¼ cup diet margarine
2 tablespoons arrowroot
1½ cups unsweetened apple
  juice
¾ cup beer

2 tablespoons white vinegar
Non-nutritive sweetener
  equivalent to 2 table-
  spoons brown sugar
½ cup raisins

Melt margarine and stir in arrowroot; gradually add apple juice and
beer, stirring constantly. Add remaining ingredients; cook over low
heat, stirring, until sauce is smooth and slightly thickened. Serve
over hot or cold tongue.

TARTAR SAUCE

Exchanges per serving: 2 tablespoons = ½ Fat
Calories per serving: 20   Yield: ½ cup

¼ cup imitation mayon-
  naise
2 tablespoons dill pickle,
  chopped

1 tablespoon diet margarine
2 tablespoons parsley,
  minced
1 teaspoon lemon juice
¼ teaspoon salt

Mix all ingredients together; chill before serving. Store in refrigerator.

CELERY AND TOMATO SAUCE

Exchanges per serving: ½ cup = ½ Fat, 1 Vegetable
Calories per serving: 32   Yield: 2 cups

1 tablespoon green pepper,
  minced fine
2 tablespoons dried onion
1 cup celery, sliced thin
1 tablespoon diet margarine
1 scant cup tomato sauce

½ teaspoon sesame seeds,
  crushed fine
¼ teaspoon lemon pepper
Dash of salt
Dash of black pepper
¼ teaspoon garlic salt

Sauté pepper, onion, and celery in margarine until golden and wilted. Add remaining ingredients; boil gently about 30 minutes. Serve over fish or meat.

SPAGHETTI SAUCE

Exchanges per serving: 1 cup = ½ Fat, 2 Vegetable
Calories per serving: 73 (sauce only)　　　　　Yield: 10 cups

½ cup celery, chopped fine
1½ cups onion, chopped fine
8 cups tomatoes
1 cup tomato sauce
½ teaspoon thyme
½ teaspoon marjoram
⅛ teaspoon celery salt

Dash of garlic salt
¼ teaspoon rosemary
1 teaspoon oregano
½ teaspoon basil
¼ teaspoon salt
Dash of pepper

Sauté celery and onion in margarine until golden and wilted; add remaining ingredients. Cover and bring to a boil. Uncover and boil gently until sauce is thick. Use for noodles, spaghetti, macaroni, or meat.

RAISIN SAUCE

Exchanges per serving: 2 tablespoons = ½ Fruit
Calories per serving: 24　　　　　　　　Yield: 1½ cups

Non-nutritive sweetener
　equivalent to ¾ cup brown
　sugar
1½ tablespoons arrowroot
1½ cups broth (preferably
　tongue)

¼ cup vinegar
½ cup golden raisins
1 lemon, sliced thin

Mix sweetener and arrowroot in top of double boiler; add broth gradually, stirring constantly. Add remaining ingredients. Cook until raisins are plump and mixture thick, stirring constantly. Serve hot with ham or tongue.

CHINESE MUSTARD

Exchanges per serving: 1 tablespoon = ¼ Fat
Calories per serving: 16   Yield: ½ cup

⅓ cup dry mustard
1 tablespoon safflower oil
Non-nutritive sweetener
    equivalent to 1 tea-
    spoon sugar

½ teaspoon seasoned salt
2 teaspoons flat beer or
    wine

Mix all ingredients until smooth; serve in small dipping bowl.

APPLE-CRANBERRY RELISH

Exchanges per serving: ¼ cup = 1 Fat, 1 Fruit
Calories per serving: 74   Yield: 1¾ cups

½ cup apples, diced
2 cups fresh cranberries,
    chopped fine
¼ cup white raisins,
    chopped fine

¼ cup walnuts, chopped
    fine
Non-nutritive sweetener
    equivalent to 1 cup sugar
½ teaspoon lemon juice

Combine all ingredients, mixing well. Chill overnight in refrigerator.

LOW-CALORIE TOPPING WHIP

Exchanges per serving: ¼ cup = None
Calories per serving: 9   Yield: 3½ cups

½ cup nonfat dry milk
½ cup ice water
2 tablespoons fresh
    lemon juice

Non-nutritive sweetener
    equivalent to ¼ cup
    sugar

Place bowl and beaters in refrigerator for about two hours. Mix
nonfat milk powder and ice water in chilled bowl; beat with mixer
until soft peaks form. Add juice and sweetener; beat again until
mixture forms stiff peaks.

CUSTARD SAUCE FOR SHORTCAKE
(High Cholesterol)

Exchanges per serving: 1 tablespoon = trace Nonfat Milk
Calories per serving: 9   Yield: 2½ cups

2 cups nonfat milk	½ tablespoon arrowroot
2 eggs	¼ teaspoon salt
Non-nutritive sweetener	1 teaspoon vanilla extract
equivalent to 1½ cups	1 teaspoon almond extract
sugar	

Scald milk in saucepan. Beat eggs, sweetener, arrowroot, and salt in small bowl; gradually add scalded milk. Return mixture to saucepan; cook over low heat, stirring constantly, until mixture coats a spoon and is slightly thickened. Remove from heat; beat in vanilla and almond extracts. Chill until ready to use.

CHERRY GLAZE

Exchanges per serving: ½ cup = 1 Fruit
Calories per serving: 37   Yield: 3 cups

2 cups sour red cherries,	1 teaspoon arrowroot
water-packed, pitted;	1 tablespoon lemon juice
reserve liquid	¼ teaspoon almond extract
Non-nutritive sweetener	Drop of red vegetable food
equivalent to 2 table-	coloring (optional)
spoons sugar	

Mix ½ cup liquid from cherries with sweetner and arrowroot; stir to make smooth paste. Cook, stirring constantly, until thick and smooth. Add cherries, lemon juice, and almond extract. Allow to cool at room temperature. May be used over dietetic ice cream and on pineapple cheese pie, among other desserts.

LEMON SAUCE

Exchanges per serving: 5 tablespoons = 1 Fat
Calories per serving: 31   Yield: 1 cup

¾ tablespoon arrowroot
Non-nutritive sweetener
 equivalent to ½ cup
 sugar
⅛ teaspoon salt
1 cup boiling water
2 tablespoons diet
 margarine

1½ tablespoons lemon juice
1½ teaspoons lemon rind,
 grated fine
Dash of anise seed,
 crushed fine
Dash of nutmeg
Dash of cloves

Combine arrowroot, sweetener, and salt in saucepan; add boiling water slowly, stirring to avoid lumps. Simmer and stir until thick; remove from heat. Stir in margarine and remaining ingredients. Use for cake fillings and over bread puddings and custards.

CUSTARD SAUCE

Exchanges per serving: ½ cup = ¾ Lean Meat, ⅓ Nonfat Milk
Calories per serving: 62   Yield: 4 servings

1 whole egg plus 2 egg
 yolks
Non-nutritive sweetener
 equivalent to 3 table-
 spoons sugar

⅛ teaspoon salt
1½ cups nonfat milk
1 teaspoon vanilla extract

Beat 1 egg and 2 yolks together in saucepan (reserve 2 extra whites, covered in refrigerator, for use another time). Blend in sweetener and salt; gradually stir in nonfat milk. Place over low heat, stirring constantly, until mixture thickens slightly and coats a metal spoon. Remove from heat; stir in vanilla; chill. (Sauce will thicken more during chilling.)

POLLY'S CUSTARD SAUCE

Exchanges per serving: ½ cup = ½ Lean Meat, ½ Nonfat Milk
Calories per serving: 60   Yield: 3½ cups

3 cups nonfat milk
Non-nutritive sweetener
    equivalent to ½ cup
    sugar

1 tablespoon arrowroot
½ cup egg yolks
1 teaspoon almond extract

Combine nonfat milk and sweetener in top of double boiler; heat. Mix arrowroot and egg yolks; beat well. Add small amount of hot mixture to egg mixture; blend. Gradually blend egg mixture into milk and cook over simmering water, stirring constantly, until mixture is slightly thickened (about 15 minutes). Remove from heat; pour at once into heatproof bowl. Stir in almond extract; place in refrigerator to chill. (Sauce will thicken more as it chills.)

ORANGE SAUCE

Exchanges per serving: ¼ cup = ½ Fruit
Calories per serving: 22   Yield: 2 cups

Non-nutritive sweetener
    equivalent to 1 cup sugar
¼ teaspoon salt
1 tablespoon arrowroot
1 cup orange juice

¼ cup lemon juice
¾ cup boiling water
1 tablespoon diet margarine
1 teaspoon grated orange
    peel
1 teaspoon grated lemon
    peel

Combine sweetener, salt, and arrowroot; stir in orange and lemon juices, and boiling water. Boil 1 minute, stirring constantly. Remove from heat; stir in margarine and orange and lemon peels. Serve over hot cake or pudding.

SAUCE ROYALE

Exchanges per serving: ½ cup = 1 Fat
Calories per serving: 34   Yield: 4 servings

1 tablespoon arrowroot
½ teaspoon nutmeg
½ teaspoon cinnamon
⅛ teaspoon allspice
4 tablespoons cold water

2 cups boiling water
Dash of salt
Non-nutritive sweetener
  equivalent to 1 cup sugar
2 tablespoons diet
  margarine

Dissolve arrowroot in cold water; add spices. Add mixture to boiling water. Stir, bring to simmer; add salt, sweetener, and margarine. Use hot for custards.

SAUCE CHERRIE

Exchanges per serving: ½ cup = 1 Fruit
Calories per serving: 52   Yield: 2 cups

1 teaspoon arrowroot
2 cups water-packed
  cherries, undrained
½ teaspoon almond extract

1 teaspoon vanilla extract
Non-nutritive sweetener
  equivalent to ½ cup
  sugar

Combine arrowroot and cherries; bring to boil and simmer 5–6 minutes. Remove from heat; add extracts and sweetener. Serve slightly warm over dietetic ice cream, custards, and the like.

CHOCOLATE SAUCE

Exchanges per serving: 1 tablespoon = 2 Fat
Calories per serving: 93   Yield: 1 cup

8 ounces unsweetened
  chocolate
¼ cup water

Non-nutritive sweetener
  equivalent to ¼ cup
  sugar
½ cup nondairy whipped
  topping

Combine chocolate, water, and sweetener. Melt over hot water in double boiler. Stir until smooth; remove from heat; cool. Blend in whipped cream. Serve either hot or cold.

CITRUS FRUIT SAUCE

Exchanges per serving: ¼ cup = ¾ Fat
Calories per serving: 31   Yield: 1 cup

Non-nutritive sweetener
    equivalent to ½ cup
    sugar
2 teaspoons arrowroot
⅛ teaspoon salt
1 cup boiling water
2 tablespoons diet mar-
    garine, melted

1½ tablespoons fruit juice
    (grapefruit, lemon, or
    orange)
1½ teaspoons grated fruit
    rind
Dash of nutmeg

Combine sweetener, arrowroot, and salt in a saucepan. Stir in boiling water until smooth; stir and simmer until clear and thick. Stir in remaining ingredients.

HAWAIIAN CURRY SAUCE

Exchanges per serving: ½ cup = 3 Fat, ½ Fruit,
                        ½ Nonfat Milk
Calories per serving: 212 (sauce only)   Yield: 2 cups

¼ cup safflower oil
1 onion, minced
2 apples, peeled and diced
2½ teaspoons arrowroot
2 cups nonfat milk or
    coconut milk

1 teaspoon garlic salt
1 teaspoon salt
1 teaspoon ground ginger
3 tablespoons soy sauce
1 to 3 teaspoons curry
    powder (to taste)

Heat oil. Add onion and apples; cover and cook 10 minutes, stirring occasionally. Add arrowroot and stir until smooth; add nonfat milk or coconut milk with remaining ingredients, stirring constantly until mixture thickens and boils. Reduce heat to very low; cover and cook 20 minutes. Mix sauce with 2 cups cooked seafood, chicken, or meat and serve on steamed rice, or as called for in recipe.

MAPLE-FLAVORED SAUCE

Exchanges per serving: ¼ cup = ½ Fat, ½ Nonfat Milk
Calories per serving: 60   Yield: 1¾ cups

¼ cup diet margarine
1 tablespoon arrowroot
Non-nutritive sweetener
    equivalent to 1 cup
    sugar

½ cup water
1 cup nonfat evaporated
    milk
1½ teaspoons maple
    flavoring

Melt margarine. Blend in arrowroot; add sweetener, water, and milk. Cook over medium heat, stirring constantly until thick. Remove from heat; add maple flavoring and chill.

VEGETABLES

See Packaged Food tables for additional suggestions.

JUICES

Tomato Juice, 6 ounces . . . . .35 calories
Vegetable Cocktail Juice, 6 ounces . . . . .35 calories

EGGPLANT, PEPPER, AND MUSHROOMS

Exchanges per serving: 1 cup = ½ Fat, 2 Vegetable
Calories per serving: 76   Yield: 12 cups

1 eggplant, cut and diced
    into squares (4 cups)
⅓ cup oil
½ cup water
2 large green peppers,
    cored and diced
1 cup sliced mushrooms,
    drained

2 cups tomatoes, peeled
    and diced
1 clove garlic, minced
    very fine
1 teaspoon salt
Non-nutritive sweetener
    equivalent to 1 tea-
    spoon sugar
½ teaspoon pepper

Place squares of eggplant (unpeeled) into frying pan with 3 table-spoons heated oil. Sauté over medium heat 2 minutes, turning often. Add 2 tablespoons water; cover and cook, adding water, 2 table-spoons at a time, as it is absorbed. Turn eggplant occasionally until tender (about 10 minutes). Remove from pan into bowl. Add balance of oil to pan; sauté peppers about 10 minutes; add mushrooms and heat until soft; add to eggplant. Add remaining ingredients to pan; simmer until mixture becomes a thick sauce; pour over eggplant. Mix lightly.

EGGPLANT DELIGHT

Exchanges per serving: 1 cup = ⅓ Fat, 1½ Vegetable
Calories per serving: 48   Yield: 6 cups

1 onion, sliced thin
¼ green pepper, chopped
   fine
2 tablespoons diet
   margarine

3 cups eggplant, peeled,
   cubed
2 cups tomatoes
½ teaspoon salt
⅛ teaspoon pepper

Sauté onion and pepper in margarine in medium skillet, tightly covered, until soft. Add eggplant cubes, tomatoes, salt, and pepper; cover. Simmer until eggplant is tender (about 10 minutes).

DORIS' CREAMED MUSHROOMS

Exchanges per serving: ½ cup = 1 Fat, 1 Vegetable
Calories per serving: 64   Yield: 6 cups

1 envelope dry cream of
   mushroom soup mix
2 cups water
4 cups fresh mushrooms

3 tablespoons diet mar-
   garine
1 tablespoon lemon juice
Dash of salt
Dash of pepper

Add soup mix to water; boil gently, stirring now and then, for about 10 minutes. Sauté mushrooms in margarine in large skillet until browned on all sides. Pour soup and lemon juice over mushrooms. Season.

CREAMED SPINACH

Exchanges per serving: ⅔ cup = 1 Fat, 1 Vegetable,
                          ¼ Nonfat Milk
Calories per serving: 89   Yield: 2 cups

1 clove garlic, minced fine
1 tablespoon diet margarine
1¼ cups frozen spinach,
   chopped

½ teaspoon salt
⅛ teaspoon pepper
½ teaspoon arrowroot
½ cup nonfat milk

Sauté garlic in margarine until brown; discard garlic. Add spinach, which has been thoroughly thawed, salt, and pepper; separate spinach with a fork. Cover tightly. Cook over low heat until spinach is tender and liquid has evaporated (about 4–5 minutes). Form a smooth paste of arrowroot and milk; add to cooked spinach. Heat, stirring constantly, until thick and smooth.

GOURMET SPINACH

Exchanges per serving: scant ½ cup = 1 Fat, 1 Vegetable
Calories per serving: 64   Yield: 2¾ cups

1 cup mushrooms, thinly
  sliced
1 onion chopped fine
1 clove garlic, minced
1 tablespoon diet margarine

1¼ cups frozen spinach,
  chopped
½ cup imitation sour cream
  or sour half-and-half
1 teaspoon salt
⅛ teaspoon pepper

Sauté mushrooms, onion, and garlic in margarine until onion is golden. Place spinach on top of mushroom mixture; cover, stirring now and then. Cook until spinach is heated through (8–9 minutes). Stir in sour cream, salt, and pepper.

GREEN BEAN SPECIAL

Exchanges per serving: ¾ cup = 1 Vegetable
Calories per serving: 18   Yield: 4½ cups

1 wafer-thin strip bacon
1 clove garlic, minced fine
¼ cup onion, chopped fine
2 tablespoons green pepper,
  chopped fine
1 cup tomatoes, chopped

2½ cups green beans
1¼ teaspoons salt
⅛ teaspoon pepper
½ teaspoon oregano
⅓ cup water

Cook, drain, and crumble wafer-thin strip of bacon. Pour out all fat, leaving a light coating in pan. Sauté garlic, onion, and pepper until onion is golden. Stir in remaining ingredients; cover. Cook gently until beans are tender (about 15 minutes).

GREEN BEANS DE LUXE

Exchanges per serving: ¾ cup = ½ Fat, 1 Vegetable
Calories per serving: 38   Yield: 4½ cups

4 cups canned green beans,
  undrained
¼ cup mint flakes, dried
Non-nutritive sweetener
  equivalent to 1 table-
  spoon sugar

2 tablespoons diet
  margarine
Dash of salt
Dash of pepper

Heat beans and mint flakes with sweetener to boiling point; drain. Stir in remaining ingredients.

ASPARAGUS WITH HERBS

Exchanges per serving: 1 serving = ½ Fat, 1 Vegetable
Calories per serving: 32   Yield: 3 servings

1¼ cups asparagus
1 tablespoon diet margarine
½ teaspoon salt
¼ cup water

2 tablespoons chives,
  chopped
Dash of seasoned salt
Dash of pepper

Place margarine, salt, water, and chives in skillet; cover tightly. Bring to boil. Add asparagus; cover and boil gently until asparagus is tender. Sprinkle with seasoned salt and pepper.

PEAS AND LETTUCE

Exchanges per serving: 1 serving = 1 Fat, ½ Bread, 1 Vegetable
Calories per serving: 80   Yield: 4 servings

1¼ cups frozen peas
1 cup lettuce, coarsely torn

4 tablespoons diet mar-
  garine (or omit mar-
  garine and delete fat
  exchange)

Cook peas in boiling salted water until tender (5–6 minutes); add lettuce and simmer until wilted and transparent. Drain. Toss with margarine.

BEETS WILLIAM-STYLE

Exchanges per serving: 1 serving = 1 Vegetable
Calories per serving: 40   Yield: 4 servings

Non-nutritive sweetener
  equivalent to 2 table-
  spoons sugar
½ teaspoon salt

½ teaspoon pepper
¾ teaspoon arrowroot
2 cups sliced beets
2 tablespoons lemon juice

Mix sweetener, salt, pepper, and arrowroot. Drain liquid from beets, saving ⅓ cup. Stir the ⅓ cup liquid with lemon juice and drained beets into sweetened mixture. Boil until sauce thickens and beets are heated, stirring constantly.

TOMATOES WITH CHEESE TOPPING

Exchanges per serving: 1 serving = ¼ Meat, 1 Vegetable
Calories per serving: 37   Yield: 4 servings

2 tomatoes, peeled and
  halved
½ teaspoon thyme
2 tablespoons American
  cheese, finely grated

2 tablespoons seasoned
  dried bread crumbs
½ teaspoon salt
⅛ teaspoon pepper

Preheat oven to 375°F. Place tomatoes, cut side up, in baking pan; top each half with a mixture of remaining ingredients. Bake until tomatoes are tender and cheese melts (about 20 minutes). Put baking pan under broiler for the last minute or so, to brown tops.

CELERY AND CARROTS (WITH HORSERADISH)

Exchanges per serving: 1 serving = ½ Fat, 1 Vegetable
Calories per serving: 32   Yield: 6 servings

2 cups carrots, cut into
  ½" slices
⅔ cup celery, cut into
  ½" pieces
½ cup water

1½ teaspoons prepared
  horseradish
½ teaspoon salt
2 tablespoons diet
  margarine

Scrape carrots before slicing; remove any strings from celery and slice. Place carrots and celery in saucepan with water, horseradish, and salt; cover tightly and boil until tender (about 20 minutes). Drain and add margarine.

SWEET CARROTS

Exchanges per serving: ⅔ cup = 1 Fat, 1 Vegetable
Calories per serving: 60   Yield: 2 cups

1 tablespoon diet margarine
2 tablespoons water
½ teaspoon salt
⅛ teaspoon pepper
Non-nutritive sweetener
  equivalent to ½ tea-
  spoon sugar

2 tablespoons parsley,
  snipped fine
2 cups carrots, scraped
  and sliced thin

Melt margarine; add remaining ingredients. Cover; simmer gently about 10 minutes, stirring occasionally.

GINGERED CARROTS

Exchanges per serving: ½ cup = ½ Fat, 1 Vegetable
Calories per serving: 36   Yield: 2½ cups

2 cups carrots, cut julienne
½ cup water
½ teaspoon Mei Yen
  seasoning
½ teaspoon ginger

Non-nutritive sweetener
  equivalent to ½ tea-
  spoon sugar
2 tablespoons diet
  margarine

Cook carrots in water seasoned with Mei Yen powder; add ginger, sweetener; when carrots are tender, add margarine. Continue to cook 3–4 minutes, stirring gently.

CARROTS WITH ORANGE

Exchanges per serving: ½ cup = ½ Fat, 1 Vegetable
Calories per serving: 45   Yield: 6 servings

Water to cover carrots
3 teaspoons salt
3 cups carrots, scraped and
  thinly sliced

Non-nutritive sweetener
  equivalent to 1 table-
  spoon sugar
2 tablespoons diet
  margarine
1 orange, cut into sections

Place 2 teaspoons salt in water; gently boil carrots until tender. Add remaining salt, sweetener, margarine, and oranges. Heat slowly and gently.

DELIGHTFUL CARROTS

Exchanges per serving: 1 serving = 1½ Fat, 1 Vegetable
Calories per serving: 82   Yield: 4 servings

6 carrots, peeled and cut
  into 3″ strips
4 tablespoons diet
  margarine

1 tablespoon lemon juice
⅛ teaspoon celery seed
½ teaspoon salt
2 tablespoons water

Preheat oven to 350°F. Arrange carrots in small baking dish. Melt margarine and combine with remaining ingredients. Pour over carrots. Cover and bake about 45 minutes, or until carrots are tender.

CARROTS WITH CHEESE

Exchanges per serving: 1 cup = ½ Lean Meat, ½ Fat, 1 Vegetable
Calories per serving: 75   Yield: 2 cups

2 cups carrots, sliced
½ cup cheese, grated—
  Neufchâtel or Parmesan

⅛ teaspoon salt
⅛ teaspoon pepper
1 tablespoon parsley flakes

Boil carrots gently in water to cover about 5 minutes; turn off heat and drain thoroughly. Return to saucepan; sprinkle with cheese, letting carrots stay over low heat until cheese melts. Sprinkle with salt and pepper and top with parsley.

SWEET AND SOUR RED CABBAGE

Exchanges per serving: 1 serving = ½ Fruit, 1 Vegetable
Calories per serving: 45   Yield: 8 servings

1 small head red cabbage   3 tablespoons fructose
½ cup water   ¼ teaspoon salt
2 teaspoons cornstarch   ½ teaspoon caraway seeds
½ cup cider vinegar

Shred cabbage; steam over rapidly boiling water 10 minutes, or until crisp-tender. Remove from heat; drain thoroughly. Dissolve cornstarch in water; add remaining ingredients; cook over medium heat until slightly thickened. Put cooked cabbage in large mixing bowl; add sauce and mix well. Use this dish with either hot or cold meat. NOTE: This recipe is provided through the courtesy of Sweet Lite Fructose.

PINEAPPLE SWEET POTATOES

Exchanges per serving: ½ cup (approximately 5 ounces) = 1 Bread,
                       ½ Fat, ½ Fruit
Calories per serving: 122   Yield: 8 servings

24 ounces (1½ lbs.) sweet   2 cups artificially sweet-
   potatoes   ened pineapple tidbits
1½ teaspoons salt   2 tablespoons diet
⅛ teaspoon pepper   margarine

Boil potatoes until tender; peel; cool slightly. Mash until smooth; stir in remaining ingredients, including syrup from pineapple tidbits. Return to stove and reheat.

BAKED POTATOES, STUFFED

Exchanges per serving: 1 potato = 1 Bread, 2 Fat
Calories per serving: 170   Yield: 8 servings

8 potatoes (4 ounces each)   1½ teaspoons salt
1 tablespoon oil   ⅛ teaspoon pepper
1½ cups sour half-and-half   2 tablespoons chives,
                                     snipped

Preheat oven to 450°F. Prick skins of potatoes with fork; lightly oil your hands and rub oil onto the potatoes. Place potatoes in oven and bake until done (about 35–40 minutes). Reduce heat to 325°F. Remove potatoes from oven; cut a thin slice from each and hollow out, being careful to leave shell intact. Mash centers in mixer with sour half-and-half, salt, pepper, and chives; refill shells, heaping high. Bake on aluminum foil until heated through and top is lightly browned (about ½ hour).

ANNE'S STUFFED BAKED POTATOES WITH CHEESE

Exchanges per serving: 1 potato = 1 Bread, 2 Fat, ¼ Lean Meat
Calories per serving: 135   Yield: 8 servings

8 potatoes (4 ounces each)	Dash of salt
5 tablespoons diet margarine	Dash of pepper
½ cup skim milk	1 cup cheese, finely grated—Mild Cheddar, American, or Neufchâtel

Preheat oven to 400°F. Bake potatoes until done (approximately 1 hour). While hot, cut tops off and scoop insides into mixing bowl (keeping the 8 shells intact). Add margarine and skim milk; beat until smooth. Add remaining ingredients and continue beating until mixed thoroughly. Refill potato shells, place on baking pan for 20 minutes, then under broiler until delicately browned.

MARGE'S STUFFED POTATOES

Exchanges per serving: 1 potato = 1 Bread, 1½ Fat
Calories per serving: 175   Yield: 6 servings

6 potatoes (4 ounces each)	3½ tablesppons Parmesan cheese, grated
1 teaspoon salt	½ teaspoon pepper
1 tablespoon chives, finely chopped	1 tablespoon imitation sour cream or sour half-and-half
2 tablespoons bacon bits	
½ cup diet margarine	Dash of paprika

Preheat oven to 400°F. Grease, using ''Pam'' or similar coating, then bake potatoes until soft. Cut in half lengthwise; spoon out centers into mixing bowl while hot, saving skins. Add remaining ingredients except paprika; mix about 3 minutes at medium speed of electric mixer. Place mixture in potato skins. Sprinkle lightly with paprika and brown in oven about 4 minutes.

POLLY'S CREAMED POTATOES

Exchanges per serving: ¾ cup = 1 Bread, ½ Nonfat Milk
Calories per serving: 120   Yield: 8 servings

8 potatoes (4 ounces each), peeled and cubed
1 onion, thinly sliced
1 cup celery, thinly sliced
¾ tablespoon chervil
2 teaspoons salt
⅛ teaspoon pepper

2½ cups nonfat milk
2 tablespoons diet margarine
2 tablespoons water
1½ teaspoons arrowroot
2 tablespoons dried parsley

Mix all ingredients except water, arrowroot, and parsley in saucepan; cook until potatoes are tender (20–25 minutes). Mix arrowroot and water to make a thin paste; stir into potatoes. Cover and cook until thick and smooth, stirring occasionally. Garnish with parsley.

SUPER RICE

Exchanges per serving: Generous ½ cup = 1 Bread, 1 Fat
Calories per serving: 127   Yield: 8 servings

1 cup white rice
¼ teaspoon lemon juice
1 cup + 2 tablespoons frozen peas
Non-nutritive sweetener equivalent to 1 table-spoon sugar

1 onion, diced fine
2 tablespoons salad oil
½ teaspoon parsley flakes

Cook rice according to directions on package, but substitute lemon juice for butter. Cook peas; add sweetener. Sauté onion in oil until wilted and golden. Add peas and onion to rice. Garnish with parsley.

BREADS

EASY RAISIN BREAD

Exchanges per serving: 1 slice = 1 Bread, ½ Fat
Calories per serving: 104   Yield: 15 slices

½ cup quick-cooking oatmeal
1 teaspoon baking powder
2 cups biscuit mix
¼ teaspoon salt
½ cup white raisins

Non-nutritive sweetener equivalent to ¾ cup + 1 tablespoon sugar
1 egg, well beaten
1¼ cups nonfat milk

Preheat oven to 350°F. Combine dry ingredients; mix remaining ingredients and add to dry ingredients; blend well. Pour into well-greased 1-quart round casserole. Bake until done (about one hour). Cool ten minutes before turning out on rack.

RAISIN BREAD

Exchanges per serving: 1½″ slice = 1 Bread, 1 Fat, ½ Fruit, ½ Lean Meat
Calories per serving: 174   Yield: 16 servings

3 cups flour
3½ teaspoons baking powder
Non-nutritive sweetener equivalent to ¾ cup sugar
1½ teaspoons salt
⅓ cup diet margarine

2 teaspoons orange peel, grated
2 eggs
1 cup nonfat milk
1 cup white raisins, chopped
½ cup nuts, chopped fine

Preheat oven to 350°F. Sift dry ingredients; add margarine, orange peel, eggs, and nonfat milk. Mix until blended; stir in raisins and nuts. Place in well-greased 9 × 5 × 3 loaf pan. Bake 1 hour and 15 minutes or until loaf tests done. Remove from pan; cool and store 12 hours before slicing.

BARBARA'S BANANA BREAD

Exchanges per serving: ¾″ slice = 1 Bread, ½ Fat, ⅓ Fruit
Calories per serving: 110   Yield: 12 slices

¼ teaspoon baking soda
½ teaspoon salt
1¾ cups flour
2 teaspoons baking powder
Non-nutritive granulated
  sweetener equivalent to
  1 cup sugar

¼ cup diet margarine,
  melted
1 egg, well beaten
1 teaspoon almond extract
2 bananas, well mashed

Preheat oven to 350°F. Sift dry ingredients together. Combine margarine, egg, and almond extract; add to first mixture, stirring until flour is moistened. Fold in mashed bananas. Turn into 9″ well-greased loaf pan. Bake until done (about 1 hour).

SHORTBREAD

Exchanges per serving: 1″ × 3″ piece = ¼ Bread, 1 Fat, ⅓ Fruit
Calories per serving: 69   Yield: 36 servings

½ cup diet margarine
Non-nutritive sweetener
  equivalent to 1½ cups
  brown sugar
1 cup plus 2 tablespoons
  flour, sifted
2 eggs
1 teaspoon vanilla extract

1 teaspoon orange peel,
  grated
½ teaspoon salt
1 teaspoon baking powder
1½ cups white raisins,
  chopped
1 cup nuts, chopped fine

Preheat oven to 375°F. Mix margarine, half the sweetener, and 1 cup flour together to fine crumbs; press firmly in the bottom of a 13 × 9 × 2 pan. Bake 10 minutes. Meanwhile beat eggs until fluffy; beat in remaining sweetener, vanilla, and orange peel. Add remaining flour, salt, and baking powder; mix well. Stir in raisins and nuts; place mixture over crust, which has been slightly cooled. Place entire mixture in oven; bake another 30 minutes. Cool slightly before cutting.

"SEEDED" BREAD

Exchanges per serving: 1 slice = 1 Bread, ½ Fat
Calories per serving: 80   Yield: 1 slice

1 slice bread
1 teaspoon diet margarine
¼ teaspoon celery seeds

½ teaspoon poppy seeds
¼ teaspoon sesame seeds
Dash of garlic salt

Spread bread with margarine. Sprinkle with combination of seeds, then garlic salt. Place under broiler until edges of bread are brown and margarine melted. Serve hot or cool (at room temperature).

DATE AND NUT BREAD

Exchanges per serving: 1 slice = 1 Bread, 1 Fat, 1 Fruit
Calories per serving: 156   Yield: 2 loaves
                                                   (16 slices each)

4 cups dates, pitted
2 cups nuts, coarsely
   chopped
2 cups boiling water
2¾ cups flour
1½ teaspoons baking soda
1 teaspoon salt

½ cup diet margarine,
   softened
Non-nutritive sweetener
   equivalent to 1¼ cups
   brown sugar, firmly
   packed
2 eggs
1 teaspoon vanilla extract

Preheat oven to 350°F. Cut dates into small pieces with scissors; add nuts and boiling water. Allow to cool to room temperature (about 45 minutes). Sift flour with baking soda and salt. On high speed of mixer beat margarine with sweetener, eggs, and vanilla until smooth. Add date mixture; mix well. Add flour mixture; beat with a wooden spoon until well combined. Place in 2 well-greased 9 × 5 loaf pans. Bake 70 minutes or until tester inserted in center of bread comes out clean. Cool 10 minutes in pan, then on wire rack until room temperature.

PRUNE BREAD

Exchanges per serving: 1 slice = 2 Bread, 1 Fat, 1½ Fruit
Calories per serving: 254   Yield: 12 slices

2 cups dried prunes	1 teaspoon salt
1½ cups boiling water	2 teaspoons baking soda
3 cups flour	2 eggs
Non-nutritive sweetener equivalent to 1½ cups sugar	4 tablespoons salad oil

Preheat oven to 325°F. Soak prunes in cold water for two hours. Drain, then pit and chop prunes. Add boiling water; let stand 5 minutes. Sift flour, sweetener, salt, and baking soda; add prune mixture. Beat; beat in eggs, then salad oil. Pour into two greased 8½ × 4½ × 2½ loaf pans and bake for 1 hour. Remove from pans and cool on wire rack.

CORNBREAD

Exchanges per serving: 1 square = 1½ Bread, 1 Fat
Calories per serving: 145   Yield: 9 squares

1¼ cups flour	1 teaspoon salt
¾ cup yellow cornmeal	1 egg
Non-nutritive sweetener equivalent to 2 tablespoons sugar	⅔ cup nonfat milk
4½ teaspoons baking powder	⅓ cup nonfat diet margarine, melted

Preheat oven to 425°F. Sift first five ingredients into small bowl. Beat egg well; stir in milk and margarine. Pour into flour mixture all at once; stir until flour is just moistened (mixture will be lumpy). Pour into well-greased 8″ square cake pan. Spread evenly; bake until bread comes away from edges of pan (about 30 minutes). Cut into nine equal squares.

DATE BREAD

Exchanges per serving: 1 slice = 1 Bread, ¼ Fat, ½ Fruit
Calories per serving: 98   Yield: 34 slices

3 cups flour, sifted
1½ teaspoons salt
½ teaspoon ground cloves
½ teaspoon nutmeg
4½ teaspoons baking
   powder
1 teaspoon mace
½ teaspoon allspice

2 dozen dates, chopped well
1 cup nonfat milk
Non-nutritive sweetener
   equivalent to 1½ cups
   sugar
2 eggs, well beaten
¼ cup diet margarine,
   melted

Preheat oven to 350°F. Sift first seven ingredients together. Add dates; mix nonfat milk, sweetener, eggs, and margarine; add to first mixture. Pour into well-greased 9 × 5 × 3 loaf pan. Bake 1 hour and 15 minutes.

BUTTERMILK BISCUITS WITH SEEDS

Exchanges per serving: 1 biscuit = 1½ Fat, 1 Bread
Calories per serving: 150   Yield: 24 biscuits

4 cups flour
4 teaspoons baking powder
½ teaspoon baking soda
2 teaspoons salt

2 tablespoons seeds (such
   as sesame, caraway)
1½ cups buttermilk
⅔ cup safflower oil

Preheat oven to 350°F. Sift flour, baking powder, baking soda, and salt into bowl; add seeds. Add buttermilk to oil but do not stir together; pour all at once over dry ingredients. Mix with fork to make soft dough. Turn dough onto floured board; knead lightly until smooth; flatten slightly. Cover with sheet of waxed paper; roll to a 6 × 8 rectangle about ¼″ thick; remove paper. Cut into 2″ squares. Bake until brown.

JOAN'S BISCUITS

Exchanges per serving: 1 biscuit = 1 Bread, ½ Fat
Calories per serving: 94   Yield: 16 buiscuits

2 cups flour   ¼ cup diet margarine
1 teaspoon salt   ¾ cup nonfat milk
3 teaspoons baking powder

Preheat oven to 450°F. Sift flour, salt, and baking powder. Cut in
margarine until well mixed with first ingredients; add milk. Knead
several times; roll out on lightly floured board until about ½″ thick.
Cut with biscuit cutter or inverted glass, or drop by spoonfuls. Place
on well-greased heavy-duty aluminum foil or cookie sheet. Bake
until browned (13–14 minutes).

CORNMEAL BERRY MUFFINS

Exchanges per serving: 1 muffin = 1 Bread, 1 Fat
Calories per serving: 94   Yield: 15 muffins

⅓ cup diet margarine,   1¼ cups cornmeal
   melted   ¾ cup flour
Non-nutritive sweetener   2½ teaspoons baking
   equivalent to ⅓ cup   powder
   sugar   ¼ teaspoon salt
¼ cup water   ¾ cup nonfat milk
2 eggs   ⅔ cup berries (e.g., blue-
                                    berries, blackberries)

Preheat oven to 400°F. Beat together margarine, sweetener, water,
and eggs; stir in cornmeal. Sift flour, baking powder, and salt. Stir ¼
of this into first mixture with ¼ of the milk. Repeat until used. Wash
and drain berries; fold gently into batter. Place about 4 tablespoons in
each well-greased muffin cup. Bake until brown and separated from
edge of cups (about 20 minutes).

BERRY MUFFINS

Exchanges per serving: 1 muffin = 1 Bread, ½ Fat
Calories per serving: 104   Yield: 12 muffins

2 cups biscuit mix
Non-nutritive sweetener
  equivalent to ¼ cup +
  2 tablespoons sugar
1 cup unflavored yogurt

1 egg
1 cup berries (e.g., blueberries, blackberries)
2 teaspoons lemon peel,
  grated

Preheat oven to 425°F. Grease a 12-muffin (2½") tin. Combine mix
and sweetener equivalent to ¼ cup sugar in bowl; add yogurt. Add
egg; beat with fork until well combined. Fold berries gently into
batter with rubber spatula; place about ¼ cup batter into each muffin
cup. Combine lemon peel and remaining sweetener and mix well.
Sprinkle over batter; bake until golden brown (20 to 25 minutes).
Serve hot.

SOUR CREAM MUFFINS

Exchanges per serving: 1 muffin = 1 Bread, 2 Fat
Calories per serving: 151   Yield: 8 muffins

¼ cup diet margarine
¾ cup imitation sour cream
  or sour half-and-half
1⅓ cups all-purpose flour,
  sifted

Non-nutritive sweetener
  equivalent to ½ cup
  sugar
½ teaspoon baking soda
¼ teaspoon salt
Dash of nutmeg
1 egg, beaten

Preheat oven to 450°F. Cream margarine; add sour cream; mix well.
Sift dry ingredients. Add alternately with egg to first mixture. Spoon
into greased muffin tins; bake for 15 minutes.

MARY C'S MUFFINS

Exchanges per serving: 1 muffin = 1 Bread, 1 Fat
Calories per serving: 115   Yield: 24 muffins

½ cup diet margarine
Non-nutritive sweetener
   equivalent to ¾ cup
   sugar
3 eggs

4 cups flour
6 teaspoons baking powder
2 teaspoons salt
1½ cups nonfat milk

Preheat oven to 400°F. Cream together margarine and sweetener. Beat eggs and add. Sift flour, baking powder, and salt together; add alternately with nonfat milk to creamed mixture. Fill well-greased muffin pans ⅔ full. Bake 45 minutes. Serve hot.

LEMON MUFFINS

Exchanges per serving: 1 muffin = 1 Bread, 1½ Fat
Calories per serving: 149   Yield: 12 muffins

2 cups all-purpose flour,
   sifted
Non-nutritive sweetener
   equivalent to ½ cup
   sugar
3 teaspoons baking powder
½ teaspoon salt

⅔ cup nonfat milk
⅓ cup lemon juice
1 teaspoon lemon rind,
   grated
⅓ cup salad oil
1 egg, slightly beaten

Preheat oven to 400°F. Sift flour, sweetener, baking powder, and salt into a large bowl. Combine nonfat milk, lemon juice, lemon rind, oil, and egg; beat with a fork to mix well. Pour into dry ingredients; stir quickly with fork (do not beat—batter will be lumpy). Fill each well-greased muffin cup slightly more than half full. Bake 20–25 minutes, until golden (or until cake tester comes out clean). Remove from oven, loosen edges of muffins with spatula, and turn out.

PANCAKES

Exchanges per serving: 1 pancake = 1 Bread, ¼ Nonfat Milk
Calories per serving: 90   Yield: 10 4-inch pancakes

1¼ cups flour
2½ teaspoons baking
  powder
Non-nutritive sweetener
  equivalent to 2 table-
  spoons sugar

¾ teaspoon salt
1 egg
1¼ cups nonfat milk
2 tablespoons diet mar-
  garine, melted

Mix and sift flour, baking powder, sweetener, and salt in medium bowl. In another bowl beat egg; stir in nonfat milk and margarine; stir into flour mixture until dry ingredients are moist. Heat pan until water dropped on it "jumps" up and down. For each pancake, put about 3 tablespoons of mixture in pan; cook over low heat until bubbles appear on top and underside is nicely browned. Turn with spatula and brown other side.

WAFFLES

Exchanges per serving: 1 waffle = 1 Bread, 1 Fat
Calories per serving: 102   Yield: 10 4-inch waffles

1½ cups flour
2 teaspoons baking powder
½ teaspoon salt
2 eggs
1¼ cups nonfat milk

Non-nutritive sweetener
  equivalent to ¼ cup
  sugar
3 tablespoons diet mar-
  garine, melted

Heat waffle iron. Sift dry ingredients into bowl. In another bowl beat eggs, nonfat milk, sweetener, and margarine. Stir mixtures together until flour is moist and batter nearly smooth. Allow 4 tablespoons of batter for each 4-inch waffle.

AUNT JEANNE'S COFFEE CAKE

Exchanges per serving: 1 serving = 1½ Bread, 1½ Fat
Calories per serving: 185   Yield: 8 servings

2 cups flour
3 teaspoons baking powder
¼ teaspoon salt
⅓ cup diet margarine,
  softened
¾ cup nonfat milk
3 drops yellow food
  coloring

Non-nutritive sweetener
  equivalent to ¾ cup
  sugar
1 egg
½ teaspoon cinnamon
¼ cup bread crumbs,
  toasted

Preheat oven to 375°F. Sift flour, baking powder, and salt into small bowl. With electric beater, cut in 3 tablespoons margarine on lowest speed; then turn to medium speed for about 5 minutes until mixture is well blended and resembles small peas. Add ½ cup nonfat milk mixed with coloring and ½ cup sweetener. Continue beating on medium speed for about 1 minute; batter will be stiff. Add remaining nonfat milk; beat for a minute, then add unbeaten egg and beat one more minute. Pour into greased 8″ round cake pan. Mix remaining tablespoon margarine, cinnamon, and toasted bread crumbs and sprinkle on top of dough. Bake until cake springs back when lightly touched (about 20 minutes).

PAULA'S POPOVERS

Exchanges per serving: 1 popover = 2 Bread, 1 Fat, ½ Lean Meat
Calories per serving: 218   Yield: 8 popovers

2 cups flour
1 teaspoon salt
4 eggs

2 cups nonfat milk
6 tablespoons diet
  margarine, melted

Preheat oven to 350°F. Sift flour and salt. Beat eggs slightly; add milk and margarine; beat until blended. Gradually add dry ingredients. Grease ramekin cups well; fill about ¾ full. Bake 1 hour and 10 minutes; remove from oven. Slit each side quickly to release steam. Return to oven until brown and crisp and tops are firm. Lift out of ramekins; serve hot.

COFFEE CAKE, CHOCOLATE STYLE

Exchanges per serving: 1 half-inch slice = 2½ Bread, 1 Fat,
1 Lean Meat

Calories per serving: 202   Yield: 12 servings

⅔ cup diet margarine
Non-nutritive sweetener
  equivalent to 1 cup
  sugar
3 eggs
1 teaspoon orange peel,
  grated
1 cup imitation sour cream,
  sour half-and-half, *or*
  plain yogurt
1 teaspoon vanilla extract
¼ teaspoon salt

½ teaspoon baking soda
1½ teaspoons baking
  powder
2 cups + 2 tablespoons
  flour
1 ounce unsweetened
  chocolate
Non-nutritive sweetener
  equivalent to ½ cup
  brown sugar
1 teaspoon cinnamon
1 tablespoon diet margarine

Preheat oven to 350°F. Cream margarine and sweetener until light
and fluffy; add eggs one at a time, beating each until smooth. Mix in
orange peel, sour cream, and vanilla. Stir salt, baking soda, baking
powder, and 2 cups flour together; blend with creamed mixture
thoroughly. Place in a well-greased 10″ tube pan. Melt chocolate in
aluminum foil and swirl over batter with spoon to form ripples
through batter. Mix brown sugar substitute, cinnamon, and softened
margarine with remaining 2 tablespoons flour; sprinkle over batter.
Bake until tester inserted in center comes out clean (50–60 minutes).

STUFFING
(For Chicken, Turkey, or Meat)

Exchanges per serving: 1 cup = 2 Bread, ⅔ Fat
Calories per serving: 180   Yield: 6 servings

½ cup celery, chopped fine
½ cup onion, chopped fine
½ cup mushrooms,
  chopped fine

¼ cup diet margarine
8-ounce package herb-
  seasoned stuffing mix
1 cup boiling water

Sauté celery, onion, and mushrooms in margarine until onion is
golden. Add stuffing mix to boiling water, then toss all together. Mix
well.

SEEDED STUFFING
(For Chicken, Turkey, or Meat)

Exchanges per serving: ½ cup = 1 Bread, ½ Fat
Calories per serving: 85   Yield: 6 cups

1 onion, chopped fine
2 stalks celery, chopped
  fine
1 cup mushrooms, chopped
  fine
2 tablespoons diet
  margarine

8-ounce package stuff-
  ing mix
¼ teaspoon *each* celery,
  sesame, and poppy seeds
1 cup boiling water

Sauté onion, celery, and mushrooms in margarine until onion is
golden. Add stuffing mix and seeds to boiling water; mix all ingredients together.

MARVELOUS MARMALADE STUFFING

Exchanges per serving: ½ cup = 2 Bread, 2½ Fat
Calories per serving: 261   Yield: 3 cups

8-ounce package corn-
  bread stuffing
½ cup diet margarine,
  melted
½ cup celery, chopped fine

¼ cup onion, chopped fine
¼ cup almonds, slivered
  and chopped
½ cup dietetic marmalade

Mix all ingredients; toss lightly but thoroughly. Use to lightly stuff a
4- to 5-pound chicken.

DESSERTS: FRUITS, PUDDINGS, AND SOUFFLÉS

NOTE: Desserts really should be used infrequently—as opposed to never!

LUCY'S LUSCIOUS APRICOT SOUFFLÉ DESSERT

Exchanges per serving: 1 serving = 2 Fruit
Calories per serving: 85   Yield: 8 servings

1 cup dried apricots
Non-nutritive sweetener
   equivalent to 1¼ cups
   sugar
Water to cover

2 cups egg whites (10–12)
Dash of salt
1 cup low-calorie non-
   dairy whipped topping

Preheat oven to 300°F. Combine apricots and ¾ cup sweetener in a saucepan; add sufficient water to cover. Cook slowly until sweetener dissolves, stirring occasionally; cover pan and cook over low heat until apricots are tender and plump; drain. Retain syrup. Purée apricots. Beat egg whites, which should be at room temperature, with salt until egg whites are stiff; add remaining ½ cup sweetener. Fold in puréed apricots, mixing thoroughly. Turn into buttered tube pan. Bake 45 minutes. The soufflé will rise and become golden brown. Top with nondairy whip, to which 2 tablespoons apricot syrup have been added after whipping.

BAKED FRESH PEACHES

Exchanges per serving: 1 peach = 1 Fruit
Calories per serving: 40   Yield: 4 servings

    4 peaches
    1 teaspoon diet margarine

Non-nutritive sweetener
    equivalent to ½ cup
    sugar
1 tablespoon lemon juice

Preheat oven to 350°F. Cut about an inch of skin from each end of peach; set in a baking dish that has been well greased with margarine. Sprinkle with sweetener and lemon juice. Bake about 20 minutes; serve cold or hot, with milk or cream if desired.

2 tablespoons light cream = 45 calories
4 tablespoons nonfat milk = 23 calories

BANANA FREEZE

Exchanges per serving: 1 cup = 1½ Fruit
Calories per serving: 63   Yield: 6 cups

    3 bananas, crushed
    Non-nutritive sweetener
      equivalent to 2 table-
      spoons sugar

1 cup unsweetened orange
   juice
1 teaspoon lemon juice
¼ cup water

Combine all ingredients, mixing well. Divide mixture evenly into 6 paper cups and freeze until firm. Let stand at room temperature 5–6 minutes; peel paper cup as freeze is being eaten.

DIETETIC SPICED PEACHES

Exchanges per serving: 1 serving = 1 Fruit
Calories per serving: 40   Yield: 2 servings

    4 dietetic peach halves
    16 whole cloves

1 cup liquid from peaches

Preheat oven to 375°F. Place peaches in small baking pan, pitted side up. Stick 4 cloves in each half; pour liquid over fruit. Bake 20 minutes. Serve hot.

SUMMER FRUIT MIX

Exchanges per serving: ¾ cup = 1½ Fruit
Calories per serving: 60   Yield: 5 cups

2 cups strawberries
1 cup grapes
1 cup melon balls

1 cup blackberries
Non-nutritive sweetener
    equivalent to ¼ cup
    sugar

Wash and clean fruit; combine with sweetener; chill. This goes well topped with Custard Sauce for Shortcakes (see Index).

APPLESAUCE, UNCOOKED

Exchanges per serving: 1 cup = 2 Fruit
Calories per serving: 80   Yield: 4 cups

2 cups apples, washed,
    cored, and cubed, but
    not peeled
2 cups cold water
3 tablespoons lemon juice
Dash of cloves
Dash of ginger

¼ teaspoon nutmeg
Non-nutritive sweetener
    equivalent to 3 tea-
    spoons sugar
2 drops red vegetable food
    coloring (optional)

As you cut apples, place them in bowl with water and lemon juice. Remove ½ cup juice from bowl; to it add sweetener, spices, and half the apple cubes. Blend; then add the additional cubes gradually until all is smoothly blended. Add coloring.

SPICED FRUIT

Exchanges per serving: 1 cup = 2 Fruit
Calories per serving: 88   Yield: 5 cups

1 cup dietetic pineapple
   juice
¼ teaspoon cinnamon

2 cups dietetic pear halves
2 cups dietetic peach halves

Heat pineapple juice and cinnamon to boil; chill fruit, from which syrup has been drained; place in a bowl. Pour pineapple juice over fruit; serve at once.

WINE SAUCE WITH FRUIT

Exchanges per serving: 1 serving = 1 Fat, 2½ Fruit
Calories per serving: 149   Yield: 4 servings

4 cups apples, peeled and
   sliced (or substitute other
   fruit, such as bananas,
   peaches, pears)
2 tablespoons diet
   margarine

1 cup red wine
½ tablespoon arrowroot
Non-nutritive sweetener
   equivalent to 1 cup
   sugar
Dash of allspice

Brown apples in margarine. Add wine to arrowroot a little at a time to make a smooth paste. Add sweetener; cook over medium heat, stirring constantly, until clear and thick; add allspice. Pour over fruit slices and simmer a few minutes. Serve immediately.

HAWAIIAN FRUIT FRITTERS

Exchanges per serving: 1 fritter = ½ Bread, ½ Fruit, ¼ Lean Meat
Calories per serving: 73   Yield: 20 fritters

2 eggs
½ cup nonfat milk
½ teaspoon seasoned salt
2 cups cornflakes, finely
   crushed

2 cups fresh pineapple (or
   papaya or banana)
   (approximately ten 1"
   pieces per cup)

Preheat oven to 425°F. Beat eggs, nonfat milk, and salt together; cut fruit into inch-long pieces and dip in egg mixture; roll in cornflakes. Put on cookie sheet; bake for 5 to 10 minutes, until golden. Serve with Hot Shoyu (Soy) Sauce dip (see Index.)

POLLY'S PEAR DISH

Exchanges per serving: 1 slice = 1 Bread, 1 Fat, 1½ Fruit
Calories per serving: 180   Yield: 8 servings

½ cup water
Non-nutritive sweetener
  equivalent to 1 cup
  sugar
1 tablespoon fresh lemon
  juice
8 fresh pears, pared,
  cored, and sliced thin

8″ pie shell, unbaked
1 cup low-calorie apricot
  preserves
Dash of nutmeg
Dash of allspice

Preheat oven to 425°F. Combine water, sweetener, and lemon juice in saucepan. Add pear slices a few at a time; cook gently until tender (about 5–6 minutes). Cool a little, then drain, saving ¼ cup liquid. Place pear slices in circle in unbaked pie shell. Bake until golden brown; cool. Combine apricot preserves and reserved liquid in a saucepan; heat until bubbly, then force through sieve. Spoon over pear slices to glaze; sprinkle with nutmeg and allspice. Chill.

BAKED APPLES

Exchanges per serving: 1 apple = 1 Fruit
Calories per serving: 40   Yield: 2 servings

2 medium apples (approxi-
  mately 5 ounces each)
2 teaspoons lemon juice
Dash of nutmeg

Dash of cinnamon
Dash of allspice
4 tablespoons dietetic
  maple topping

Preheat oven to 350°F. Core apples and peel about ½ of each apple; sprinkle lemon juice over cut surfaces. Dust apple with mixture of nutmeg, cinnamon, and allspice. Fill cavity with dietetic maple topping; bake covered about 25 minutes. Remove cover and continue baking until apples are tender.

MARTI'S APPLE CRISP

Exchanges per serving: 1 serving = 1 Fat, 1 Fruit, ½ Bread,
                       ½ Lean Meat
Calories per serving: 135   Yield: 6 servings

4 apples, cored, peeled, and sliced	½ cup flour
¼ cup water	½ teaspoon cinnamon
½ teaspoon fresh lemon juice	½ teaspoon allspice
Non-nutritive sweetener equivalent to ⅔ cup sugar.	½ teaspoon salt
	3 tablespoons diet margarine
	½ cup Parmesan cheese, grated

Preheat oven to 325°F. Grease a shallow baking dish; place apple slices on bottom. Combine water, lemon juice, and sweetener; pour over apples. Combine dry ingredients; cut in margarine until mixture is the consistency of large peas; sprinkle over apples. If desired, cover with grated cheese.

DIETETIC APPLE CRUNCH

Exchanges per serving: 1 serving = ½ Bread, ½ Fat, 1 Fruit
Calories per serving: 86   Yield: 6 servings

2 slices dry bread	3 cups apples, cored and sliced
1 tablespoon diet margarine	1 tablespoon lemon juice
½ teaspoon cinnamon	¾ cup dietetic maple syrup
½ teaspoon allspice	

Preheat oven to 350°F. Make crumbs from bread and toast in oven. Mix toasted crumbs with margarine, cinnamon, and ¼ teaspoon allspice. Mix apples with lemon juice, maple syrup, and remainder of allspice; spread in well-greased shallow baking dish (approximately 8″ round). Cover with crumb mixture; bake 45 minutes, or until apple slices are tender. Serve warm.

TASTY APPLESAUCE

Exchanges per serving: 1 serving = ¼ Fruit, ¼ Lean Meat
Calories per serving: 20   Yield: 4 servings

4 teaspoons cinnamon
1 teaspoon salt
1 teaspoon vanilla
Non-nutritive sweetener
   equivalent to ¼ cup
   sugar

½ cup unsweetened apple-
   sauce
2 egg whites
Dash of allspice

Stir first five ingredients together. Place in refrigerator until chilled. Before serving, beat egg whites to form stiff peaks; fold applesauce mix into whites and sprinkle with allspice.

FRUIT CAKE PUDDING

Exchanges per serving: 1 = ⅓ Bread, ½ Lean Meat, ¼ Nonfat Milk
Calories per serving: 85   Yield: 6 servings

3 eggs, separated
1 tablespoon fresh citrus
   fruit peel, grated
¼ cup fresh citrus fruit juice
1½ cups nonfat milk

Non-nutritive sweetener
   equivalent to 6 table-
   spoons sugar
¼ cup flour, sifted
Dash of salt

Preheat oven to 325°F. Beat egg whites until stiff peaks form; set aside. Add fruit peel and juice to yolks, beating at medium speed until well blended. Add nonfat milk; beat about 1 minute at low speed. Add remaining ingredients; beat again at low speed until smooth. Fold into egg whites. Spoon into custard cups; place cups in baking pan filled with about 1″ water. Bake until lightly browned on top (about 45 minutes). Serve hot or cold.

FRUIT MOUNTAIN

Exchanges per serving: 1 = 1 Fruit, ¼ Nonfat Milk
Calories per serving: 60   Yield: 6 servings

1 envelope low-calorie
    vanilla pudding and pie
    filling mix
2 cups nonfat milk
1 teaspoon almond extract

8-ounce dietetic cherry or
    apple pie filling (Sego
    or other dietetic pie
    filling)
Cinnamon

Prepare pudding according to directions on package, using nonfat milk; add almond extract. Divide into 6 dessert glasses; cool. Top with pie filling and sprinkle with cinnamon.

LEMON PUDDING

Exchanges per serving: 1 cup = 3 Fat, 2 Lean Meat
Calories per serving: 275   Yield: 4 servings

Non-nutritive sweetener
    equivalent to 1½ cups
    sugar
½ cup diet margarine

2 tablespoons lemon peel
8 eggs
1 cup lemon juice

Combine all ingredients in top of double boiler; cook over boiling water until thick, stirring constantly. Cover and store in refrigerator until cool.

OLGA'S FRUIT FESTIVAL

Exchanges per serving: 1 serving = ½ Fat, 2½ Fruit
Calories per serving: 122   Yield: 8 servings

2 cups strawberries,
    washed and hulled
3 cups fresh peaches,
    peeled and sliced
2 cups seedless green grapes
Non-nutritive sweetener
    equivalent to ⅔ cup
    sugar

¼ cup orange curaçao
½ cup nondairy whipped
    topping
1 ounce unsweetened choc-
    olate, well grated

Sprinkle strawberries over peaches; add grapes, sweetener, and curaçao. Refrigerate overnight. Prior to serving, heat broiler. Place fruit in heatproof dessert dishes; top with whipped topping. Sprinkle top with grated chocolate; place under broiler about 30 seconds, or just until chocolate melts. Serve at once.

FRUIT WHIP

Exchanges per serving: 1 cup = ½ Nonfat Milk
Calories per serving: 45   Yield: 6 servings

1½ tablespoons unflavored
   gelatin
3 cups nonfat milk

Non-nutritive sweetener
   equivalent to ¼ cup
   sugar
2 teaspoons any fruit extract

Sprinkle gelatin over nonfat milk in saucepan; cook over low heat until gelatin dissolves. Add sweetener and fruit extract. Chill in refrigerator until mixture is consistency of egg white. Remove from refrigerator and beat at highest speed of mixer until mixture is doubled in volume (this will be very fluffy). Place in a mold and refrigerate until set. May be garnished with slice of favorite fruit, if desired.

APRICOT OR PRUNE FRUIT SNOW

Exchanges per serving: 1 serving = 1 Fruit
Calories per serving: 40   Yield: 6 servings

1 envelope lemon-flavored
   low-calorie gelatin
1 cup boiling water
1 cup unsweetened apple
   juice or apricot nectar

1 egg white
6 pieces unsweetened dried
   apricots or prunes
3 teaspoons almonds,
   slivered

Dissolve gelatin in boiling water. Add juice; cool. Chill until syrupy. Add egg white and beat until frothy. Fill 6 dessert glasses with "snow." Chill until firm; decorate each with apricot or prune and sprinkle ½ teaspoon slivered almonds over fruit.

FRUIT COCKTAIL CAKE DESSERT

Exchanges per serving: 1 section = ½ Bread, ½ Fruit,
½ Nonfat Milk

Calories per serving: 100   Yield: 10 sections

Non-nutritive sweetener
  equivalent to ½ cup
  sugar
1 tablespoon unflavored
  gelatin
¼ teaspoon salt
½ cup water
4 cups dietetic fruit cocktail
1 tablespoon lemon juice

4–5 drops almond extract
2 egg whites
1 cup nondairy whipped
  topping
10 ladyfingers, split (these
  can be made from Aunt
  Jeanne's Sponge Cake*)

Combine sweetener, gelatin, and salt; add ½ cup water and cook, stirring, over medium heat until gelatin dissolves. Chill until partially set. Drain fruit cocktail; add lemon juice and almond extract. Put gelatin mixture, egg whites, and half the fruit cocktail in a large mixing bowl. Start mixer on low speed, then turn to high and beat 10 minutes, until fluffy; chill until partially set. Fold in remaining fruit cocktail and whipped topping. Line sides of springform pan with ladyfingers. Pour filling in carefully; chill overnight. Remove sides of pan to serve.

FRUIT CRISP

Exchanges per serving: 1 serving = ½ Bread, ⅓ Fat, 1½ Fruit
Calories per serving: 101   Yield: 6 servings

4 cups fruit, peeled and
  sliced thin (apples,
  peaches, apricots)
Non-nutritive sweetener
  equivalent to ⅔ cup
  sugar
1 teaspoon fresh lemon
  juice

½ cup quick-cooking rolled
  oats
Non-nutritive sweetener
  equivalent to 2 table-
  spoons brown sugar
¼ teaspoon allspice
2 tablespoons diet
  margarine

*10 pieces of finger-shaped slices of Aunt Jeanne's Sponge Cake, each cut into quarters. See Index.

Preheat oven to 350°F. Combine fruit with half of sweetener (equivalent to ⅓ cup white sugar) and juice. Place in casserole. Combine oats, brown sugar substitute, arrowroot, allspice, and remainder of regular sugar substitute. Cut in margarine until crumbly; sprinkle evenly over fruit. Bake about 1 hour, or until tender. Serve hot or cold.

MOCHA SURPRISE

Exchanges per serving: 1 cup = None
Calories per serving: 28   Yield: 3 cups

2 envelopes unflavored
  gelatin
½ cup cold water
3 cups very strong coffee
Non-nutritive sweetener
  equivalent to ⅓ cup
  sugar

½ teaspoon vanilla
Dash of salt
3 tablespoons nondairy
  whipped topping

Soften gelatin in water in a medium-size pan. Heat, stirring constantly, until dissolved. Stir in coffee, sweetener, vanilla, and salt. Pour into an 8″ square pan; chill 2 hours. Put gelatin through potato ricer (or sieve) and spoon into 3 dessert dishes. Decorate each with 1 tablespoon nondairy whipped topping.

CHOCOLATE BISQUE CAPRI

Exchanges per serving: 2-ounce scoop = 1 Fat
Calories per serving: 45 + ice cream   Yield: 16 servings

½ cup toasted almonds,
  chopped
⅓ cup toasted coconut,
  chopped

½ teaspoon almond extract
1 quart dietetic chocolate
  ice cream, softened

Combine almonds and coconut; reserving 2 tablespoons for topping, fold remainder and almond extract quickly into ice cream. Place in small paper dessert cups and sprinkle with topping. Keep in freezer until ready to serve.

FRUIT SOUFFLÉ

Exchanges per serving: ½ cup = 1 Fruit
Calories per serving: 45   Yield: 6 servings

1 envelope unflavored
   gelatin
1 cup cold water
1 teaspoon lemon rind,
   finely grated

2 cups unsweetened, puréed
   fruit (apples, pears,
   pineapple), canned or
   cooked

Sprinkle gelatin on ½ cup water; soften a few minutes. Stir over low
heat about 3 minutes until gelatin is dissolved; add remaining water,
rind, and fruit. Chill until thick enough to mound on spoon. Beat until
very light; pour into a soufflé dish and chill until firm.

LOW-CALORIE COFFEE CREAM MOUSSE

Exchanges per serving: 1 serving = ½ Fruit, ¼ Lean Meat
Calories per serving: 61   Yield: 12 servings

2 envelopes unflavored
   gelatin
2 cups cold coffee, double
   strength
3 eggs, separated
Non-nutritive sweetener
   equivalent to ¾ cup
   sugar

1 ounce semisweet choco-
   late chips
3 tablespoons rum or
   brandy flavoring
2 cups nondairy whipped
   topping

Sprinkle gelatin over 1 cup coffee in small bowl; let soften about 5
minutes. Using a rotary beater, beat egg yolks with sweetener equivalent to ½ cup sugar until light, in the top of a double boiler. Once
light, beat in remaining coffee, chocolate chips, and softened gelatin.
Stir constantly over simmering water until chocolate is melted and
coats a metal spoon (about 10 minutes). Remove from heat; stir in
flavoring. Set top of double boiler in ice and cool, stirring often, until
mixture becomes as thick as unbeaten egg white. Beat egg whites
until soft peaks form when beaters are raised; gradually beat in
remaining sweetener, until whites are stiff and glossy. Fold gelatin

mixture into 1 cup prepared whipped topping; fold in whites gently, until well blended. Place in large mold that has been rinsed well in cold water. Place in refrigerator until firm (5–6 hours). To unmold, run knife around edge of mold; invert over serving platter. Place hot, damp cloth over mold and shake gently to release; lift off mold. Spoon 1 cup nondairy whipped topping on dessert mold before serving.

PEAR PUDDING DORIS

Exchanges per serving: 3 slices = ½ Nonfat Milk, 1 Fruit
Calories per serving: 80   Yield: 6 servings

6 tablespoons nonfat dry milk	5-ounce jar low-calorie chocolate topping
1 cup water	2 egg whites
1 envelope unflavored gelatin	1 jar unsweetened pear slices

Dissolve dry milk in ¾ cup water; on remaining ¼ cup water sprinkle gelatin to soften. Mix milk with gelatin; stir over low heat until gelatin dissolves; add chocolate topping. Cool until mixture thickens enough to mound on a spoon. Beat egg whites stiff; fold in drained pears well and line dessert dishes with 3 slices in each dish. Add chocolate mixture and chill until firm.

CAKES

LORENE'S CHEESECAKE

Exchanges per serving: 1 wedge = 2 Fat, 3 Lean Meat
Calories per serving: 130   Yield: 24 wedges

¾ cup diet margarine
Non-nutritive sweetener
  equivalent to 1¼ cups
  sugar
4 eggs
2 cups low-fat cottage
  cheese
3 tablespoons arrowroot
2 cups Neufchâtel cheese
  (2 8-ounce packages)

6 level tablespoons flour
1 cup imitation sour cream
  or sour half-and-half
½ teaspoon vanilla extract
½ teaspoon lemon juice
1 cup artificially sweetened
  crushed pineapple

Preheat oven to 350°F. Cream first two ingredients; add eggs, cottage cheese, arrowroot, Neufchâtel; blend well after each addition. Add flour, sour cream, vanilla, lemon juice, and crushed pineapple, stirring well. Pour into springform pan. Bake 2 hours. When baking, dough will rise over edge, but will not run out. Leave in oven for 2 hours with heat off; keep in refrigerator overnight.

SPICE AND MAPLE CAKE

Exchanges per serving: 1½" slice = ½ Bread, ½ Lean Meat
Calories per serving: 88   Yield: 10 servings

1 cup flour
¼ cup nonfat dry milk
1 teaspoon baking powder
1 teaspoon cinnamon
1 teaspoon nutmeg

¼ teaspoon salt
2 eggs, separated
3 egg yolks
½ cup maple flavored
  topping*
½ teaspoon cream of tartar

*Use Low-Calorie Whipped Topping and add 4 or 5 drops of maple flavoring.

Preheat oven to 325°F. Sift first six ingredients together three times. Mix five egg yolks, slightly beaten, with maple topping; beat at top speed of mixer until light and fluffy (about 10 minutes). Beat two egg whites slightly; add cream of tartar; continue to beat until whites hold a stiff peak. Fold sifted dry ingredients carefully, a small amount at a time, into egg-yolk mixture. Gently fold in egg whites; pour into 9" tube pan at once. Bake about 35 minutes, or until cake springs back when lightly touched. Invert pan and let hang until cool.

DELIGHTFUL CHEESECAKE

Exchanges per serving: 1 = ⅛ Bread, ¼ Fruit, 1 Lean Meat
Calories per serving: 80   Yield: 9 servings

4 tablespoons graham cracker crumbs	3 eggs, separated
2 envelopes unflavored gelatin	¼ cup nonfat milk
1 cup low-calorie pineapple tidbits, reserving juice	2 tablespoons lemon juice
1½ cups low-fat cottage cheese	Non-nutritive sweetener equivalent to ½ cup sugar
	1 teaspoon vanilla extract
	¼ teaspoon salt

Sprinkle 3 tablespoons graham crackers crumbs on bottom of 9" pie or cake pan; set aside. Soften gelatin in ½ cup water. Add water to pineapple juice to make ¾ cup; bring to a boil; stir in gelatin. In bowl, beat cottage cheese until nearly smooth, at highest speed on mixer (about 3–4 minutes). Add egg yolks, nonfat milk, lemon juice, sweetener, vanilla, and salt; beat well. Blend in gelatin at low speed. Chill. Stir occasionally until mixture is thick, but not set (about 1 hour). Beat whites at highest speed until soft peaks form; fold in gelatin mixture by hand. Spoon over crumbs in pan; sprinkle remaining tablespoon of crumbs over filling. Add pineapple tidbits on top; chill overnight in refrigerator.

NO-CRUST CHEESECAKE

Exchanges per serving: 1 wedge = 1½ Fat, ½ Lean Meat
Calories per serving: 100   Yield: 24 wedges

2 cups low-fat cottage
   cheese
2 cups Neufchâtel cheese,
   creamed
Non-nutritive sweetener
   equivalent to 1½ cups
   sugar
3 eggs

1½ tablespoons lemon juice
1 teaspoon vanilla extract
½ cup diet margarine,
   melted
1½ tablespoons arrowroot
3 tablespoons flour
2 cups imitation sour cream
   or sour half-and-half

Preheat oven to 325°F. Cream the cheeses together, gradually adding sweetener, beating after each addition. Add eggs, beat well; add lemon juice, vanilla and margarine. Mix arrowroot and flour with enough sour cream to make a smooth paste. Add paste and remaining sour cream to cheese mixture; blend thoroughly. Pour into greased 9″ springform pan. Bake 1 hour or longer, until firm; turn off oven. Let cake remain in oven 2 hours or longer. Place in refrigerator overnight. Serve cold.

BANANA RAISIN CAKE

Exchanges per serving: 1 slice = 1 Bread, 1 Fat, ½ Fruit
Calories per serving: 130   Yield: 18 slices

2 cups flour
1½ teaspoons baking
   powder
Non-nutritive sweetener
   equivalent to 1½ cups
   sugar
1 teaspoon baking soda
1 teaspoon salt
½ cup diet margarine

1 cup bananas (about 3),
   mashed
¼ cup nonfat milk
1 teaspoon lemon peel,
   grated
1 teaspoon vanilla extract
2 eggs
1 cup white raisins,
   chopped
½ cup nuts, chopped fine

Preheat oven to 350°F. Sift flour, baking powder, sweetener, baking soda, and salt. Add margarine, bananas, nonfat milk, lemon peel, and vanilla; beat 3 minutes on electic mixer at medium speed, scraping bowl constantly. Add eggs; beat 2 minutes more, continuing to scrape bowl frequently. Stir in raisins and nuts. Pour batter into a well-greased and lightly floured 9 × 12 × 2 pan. Bake until cake tests done. Turn out on rack to cool after 5 minutes.

CHOCOLATE CAKE

Exchanges per serving: 1 = ¾ Bread, ¾ Fat
Calories per serving: 76 (Frosting not included)   Yield: 8 servings

¾ cup flour, sifted
¼ teaspoon salt
1 teaspoon baking powder
¼ teaspoon baking soda
3 tablespoons unsweet-
    ened cocoa
¼ cup cold coffee

1 egg
Non-nutritive sweetener
    equivalent to ½ cup
    sugar
¼ cup water
1 tablespoon salad oil
1 teaspoon vanilla extract

Preheat oven to 350°F. Line an 8″ round layer cake pan with paper; grease lightly with margarine. Sift first four ingredients together; blend in cocoa and coffee. Beat egg, sweetener, water, oil, and vanilla. Stir into dry ingredients; mix until smooth. Pour batter into pan, cover with foil, and place in shallow pan of water. Bake about 30 minutes. Remove from pan; cool on cake rack. Cut crosswise, fill, and frost with desired frosting.

CHARLOTTE'S CHOCOLATE CAKE

Exchanges per serving: 1 = 1 Bread, 1 Fat, ¼ Fruit
Calories per serving: 130   Yield: 9 servings

⅓ cup diet margarine,
  softened
Non-nutritive sweetener
  equivalent to ¼ cup
  brown sugar
1 egg
Non-nutritive sweetener
  equivalent to ⅓ cup
  sugar
1⅓ cups flour

3 tablespoons unsweet-
  ened cocoa
2 teaspoons baking powder
½ teaspoon baking soda
½ cup nonfat milk
½ teaspoon vanilla extract
½ teaspoon almond extract
2 tablespoons nuts,
  chopped fine

Preheat oven to 350°F. Mix margarine, brown sugar substitute, egg, and regular sugar substitute; beat at high speed two minutes, scraping bowl occasionally. Add flour, cocoa, baking powder, baking soda, nonfat milk, and extracts; blend at low speed about 2 minutes (batter will be thick). Spread batter in a well-greased 8″ layer pan; sprinkle with nuts. Bake until tester inserted in center comes out clean.

CHOCOLATE CHIFFON CAKE WITH RUM

Exchanges per serving: 1 slice = 2 Bread, 2 Fat, ½ Lean Meat
Calories per serving: 224   Yield: 12 slices

8 eggs
½ cup cocoa
¾ cup boiling water
Non-nutritive sweetener
  equivalent to 1¾ cups
  sugar

1½ teaspoons baking soda
1¾ cups flour
½ cup soy oil
2 tablespoons rum extract
½ teaspoon cream of tartar

Preheat oven to 325°F. Let eggs reach room temperature, then separate. Combine cocoa and water in small bowl. Stir until smooth; cool. Sift sweetener, baking soda, and flour into large bowl; make well in center; add oil, egg yolks, rum extract, and cocoa mixture; beat until smooth. Add cream of tartar to egg whites; beat very stiff. Pour batter over whites; gently fold until just blended. Bake in ungreased Bundt pan (or 10″ tube pan) until straw inserted comes out clean. Cool cake completely; remove from pan. Serve plain or with nondairy whipped topping (calories and exchanges not included for topping).

LOU'S LIGHT CAKE

Exchanges per serving: 1 serving = 1½ Fat, 2 Bread
Calories per serving: 229   Yield: 10 servings

⅔ cup diet margarine
Non-nutritive sweetener
 equivalent to 2 cups
 sugar
2 teaspoons vanilla extract
2 teaspoons boiling water

1½ cups cold water
3½ cups flour, sifted
½ teaspoon salt
4 teaspoons baking powder
¾ cup (4–5) egg whites

Preheat oven to 350°F. Cream margarine and sweetener; add vanilla and boiling water; blend thoroughly. Add cold water; beat 1 minute. Sift flour and salt four times; add bit by bit, alternating with small amounts of water mixture, beating well after each addition. Beat egg whites until stiff. Sift baking powder over top of batter and fold in gently with egg whites. Bake in two well-greased and floured 10″ pans until done, or when tester comes out clean.

PAM'S QUICK LAYER CAKE

Exchanges per serving: 1 wedge = 1 Bread, 2 Fat, ½ Lean Meat
Calories per serving: 198   Yield: 12 wedges

Non-nutritive sweetener
 equivalent to 1 cup
 sugar
Dash of salt
2 cups flour
3 teaspoons baking powder
⅓ cup diet margarine

1 egg
¾ cup nonfat milk
½ teaspoon vanilla extract
½ teaspoon almond extract
1 cup pecans, chopped extra
 fine

Preheat oven to 375°F. Sift sweetener, salt, flour, and baking powder together three or four times. Cut in margarine with pastry blender or knife until mixture resembles cornmeal. Beat egg until lemon-colored and thick; add nonfat milk and extracts. Add to first mixture gradually. Add nuts and stir well. Pour into two well-greased 8″ layer pans. Bake about 25 minutes or until tester comes out clean. Cool; remove cake from pans. Cool further on wire rack.

SOUTHERN HOSPITALITY CAKE

Exchanges per serving: 1 wedge = 1 Bread, 1 Fat, ½ Fruit
Calories per serving: 142   Yield: 9 wedges

⅓ cup diet margarine, softened
Non-nutritive sweetener equivalent to ¾ cup sugar
1 egg
1⅓ cups flour
1 teaspoon baking powder
½ teaspoon baking soda
½ teaspoon orange extract
⅔ cup fresh orange juice
⅓ cup raisins
2 tablespoons nuts, chopped fine

Preheat oven to 350°F. Combine margarine, sweetener, and egg; beat 2 minutes on high speed of mixer. Scrape bowl occasionally. Add flour, baking powder, baking soda, orange extract, and juice; blend at low speed about 2 minutes (batter will be fairly thick). Stir in raisins; spread batter in a well-greased 8″ layer pan. Sprinkle nuts on top. Bake until golden brown (about 30 minutes or until tester comes out clean).

FAMILY FAVORITE CAKE

Exchanges per serving: 1 wedge = 1 Bread, 1½ Fat, ⅛ Nonfat Milk
Calories per serving: 147   Yield: 15 wedges

¾ cup diet margarine
Non-nutritive sweetener equivalent to 1½ cups sugar
4 teaspoons baking powder
½ teaspoon salt
3 cups flour
1 cup nonfat milk
1 teaspoon almond extract
¾ cup egg whites

Preheat oven to 375°F. Cream margarine and sweetener. Sift baking powder, salt, and flour. Add alternately with nonfat milk to creamed mixture; add almond extract. Beat egg whites until stiff peaks form; fold in. Pour into two well-greased 9″ layer pans. Bake about 30 minutes. Cool a few minutes; remove from pans; cool further on wire rack.

ORANGE CHIFFON CAKE

Exchanges per serving: 1½″ slice = 2 Bread, 1 Fat
Calories per serving: 160   Yield: 16 squares

8 egg whites
5 egg yolks
½ teaspoon cream of tartar
2¼ cups flour, sifted
3 teaspoons baking powder
1 teaspoon salt
Non-nutritive sweetener
   equivalent to 1½ cups
   sugar

½ cup salad oil
3 tablespoons orange peel,
   finely grated
Artificial sweetener
   equivalent to ¼ cup
   sugar added to ¾ cup
   orange juice

Preheat oven to 325°F. Bring eggs to room temperature. Add cream of tartar to egg whites; beat until they stand in peaks (stiffer than for meringue). Sift dry ingredients; make a well in center; add salad oil, egg yolks, peel, and juice-sweetener mixture; stir to blend. Beat one minute at medium speed. Add yolk-orange mixture to whites slowly, folding these together until smooth and completely mixed. Pour into an 8″ square cake pan that has been rinsed (shake out excess water). Bake until cake is pale golden brown and a cake tester comes out clean (about 30 minutes or a little more). Invert pan and cool. When cake pan is cool enough to handle (but not cold), run a knife around edges of pan; then with fingertips carefully pull cake away from edges, lifting slightly to loosen bottom. Cool on rack. Cut into serving pieces.

ORANGE CAKE

Exchanges per serving: 1 slice = 1 Bread, 1 Fat, ½ Lean Meat
Calories per serving: 142   Yield: 10 slices

1 cup flour
1½ teaspoons baking
  powder
½ teaspoon salt
¼ cup oil
4 eggs, separated

½ cup unsweetened frozen
  orange juice concentrate
Non-nutritive sweetener
  equivalent to 1½ cups
  sugar
¼ teaspoon cream of tartar

Preheat oven to 350°F. Sift flour, baking powder, and salt together. Set aside one egg yolk.* Add, in order, oil, 3 egg yolks, orange juice concentrate, and sweetener; beat until smooth. Add cream of tartar to egg whites and beat until stiff. Add egg yolk mixture to whites; fold in gently until blended, but do not overmix. Pour into 9″ tube pan; bake 35 minutes.

*Refrigerate for future use.

LOU'S CHIFFON CAKE

Exchanges per serving: 1 serving = 1½ Bread, 2 Fat
Calories per serving: 200   Yield: 12 servings

1 teaspoon salt
2¼ cups flour, sifted
3 teaspoons baking powder
½ cup salad oil
4 eggs, separated
½ cup water

Non-nutritive sweetener
  equivalent to 1½ cups
  sugar
2 teaspoons lemon rind,
  grated
1 teaspoon vanilla extract
½ teaspoon cream of tartar

Preheat oven to 325°F. Sift salt, flour, and baking powder. Add oil, well-beaten egg yolks, water, sweetener, rind, and vanilla. Beat until smooth. Beat egg whites until stiff; add cream of tartar; beat until very stiff peaks form. Gently fold batter into egg whites until just blended (do not stir). Place in ungreased 9″ tube pan. Bake until done (about 1 hour). Invert cake to cool.

MARGARET'S POUND CAKE

Exchanges per serving: 1½" slice = 2 Bread, 2 Fat, ½ Lean Meat
Calories per serving: 277   Yield: 15 servings

1 teaspoon salt
4 cups flour
½ teaspoon cream of tartar
2 cups diet margarine

Non-nutritive sweetener
  equivalent to 2 cups
  sugar
8 eggs
1 teaspoon vanilla extract
½ teaspoon allspice

Preheat oven to 325°F. Sift salt, flour, and cream of tartar, set aside. Cream margarine until fluffy; add sweetener gradually; continue to cream until very fluffy. Beat in eggs two at a time, beating well between additions; add vanilla and allspice, beating well. Add flour mixture a little at a time until well mixed. Turn batter into greased and lightly floured Bundt pan (or two 9 × 5 × 3 bread pans). Bake 1¼ to 1½ hours for Bundt cake or 1 hour for loaf cakes. Cool in pans; turn out on wire rack and cool completely. May be sprinkled with substitute confectioners' sugar.

STRAWBERRY SHORTCAKE

Exchanges per serving: 1 cake = 2 Bread, 1 Fat
                       ½ cup berries = ½ Fruit
Calories per serving: 1 cake, 190   Yield: 6 servings
berries, 20; topping, 14 per tablespoon

2 cups flour
Non-nutritive sweetener
  equivalent to 1 table-
  spoon sugar
½ teaspoon salt
3 teaspoons baking powder
4 tablespoons diet
  margarine
½ cup water

1 quart strawberries (or
  other fruit) sweetened
  with non-nutritive
  sweetener equivalent to
  1 teaspoon sugar
1 cup nondairy whipped
  topping, whipped with
  non-nutritive sweetener
  equivalent to 1 tea-
  spoon sugar

Preheat oven to 475°F. Sift flour, sweetener, salt, and baking powder; add margarine; mix thoroughly with fork. Add water to make soft dough. Roll out on floured board until about ½" thick and cut with large biscuit cutter dipped in flour, *or* half-fill large greased muffin rings that have been placed on a baking sheet. Bake 10–12 minutes. Split while hot, and fill with crushed sweetened berries. Put on tops; cover with berries and sweetened whipped topping.

MARY'S SPONGE CAKE

Exchanges per serving: 1½" slice = ½ Bread, ½ Lean Meat
Calories per serving: 66   Yield: 12 servings

1 cup flour
¼ cup nonfat dry milk
1 teaspoon baking powder
¼ teaspoon salt
3 eggs

Non-nutritive sweetener
   equivalent to 8 tea-
   spoons sugar
2 tablespoons fresh orange
   juice
1 teaspoon orange rind,
   grated
½ teaspoon cream of tartar

Preheat oven to 325°F. Sift flour, dry milk, baking powder, and salt together three times; beat 2 whole eggs and 1 yolk at top speed of mixer until quite thick and lemon-colored (about 10 minutes). Reduce speed; add sweetener gradually, then orange juice; increase speed and beat until very light and fluffy (5–6 minutes). Add rind and beat a little more. Beat remaining egg white slightly; add cream of tartar and continue beating until white holds a stiff peak. Let stand while completing next step. Very carefully fold sifted dry ingredients, a small amount at a time, into egg-sweetener mixture, using rubber spatula or wire whip. Fold in single egg white very carefully. Pour at once into 9" tube pan. (If pan has removable bottom, no need to line or grease pan; knife will help loosen cake from bottom. Otherwise, line just the bottom of pan with piece of thin waxed paper, moistened well with water to make it lie flat.) Bake about 35 minutes. Cake is done when it springs back when touched with finger. Cool in pan upside down and remove carefully.

AUNT JEANNE'S SPONGE CAKE

Exchanges per serving: ½" slice = ½ Bread, ½ Lean Meat
Calories per serving: 70   Yield: 20 servings
(does not include ice cream exchange
and calorie count)

1 cup nonfat milk	6 eggs
1¾ cups flour	Non-nutritive sweetener
2 teaspoons baking powder	equivalent to 2 cups
½ teaspoon salt	sugar
	2 teaspoons vanilla

Preheat oven to 350°F. Scald nonfat milk in small saucepan. Remove
from heat; put aside until lukewarm. Sift flour, baking powder, and
salt. Beat eggs until thick and lemon-colored; gradually add sweetener, beating, until mixture is well blended and smooth (4–5 minutes). Blend in flour mixture at low speed of mixer until smooth; add
lukewarm milk and vanilla. Continue beating until well mixed. Pour
batter into ungreased 10" tube pan; bake 50 minutes, or until tester
inserted in center of cake comes out clean. Turn cake—and cake
pan—upside down; place tube over the neck of a bottle. This allows
air to circulate around top (upside down) of cake, cooling it. Serve
with imitation strawberry ice cream.

VANILLA SPONGE ROLL

Exchanges per serving: 1 serving = ⅓ Bread, ⅔ Lean Meat
Calories per serving: 76 + 32 calories for jelly   Yield: 6 servings

4 eggs, separated	1 teaspoon baking powder
Non-nutritive sweetener	5 tablespoons potato flour
equivalent to 4 table-	1 teaspoon vanilla
spoons sugar	¼ cup dietetic jelly

Preheat oven to 325°F. Beat egg whites until stiff; add sweeteners.
Fold in beaten yolks and remaining ingredients (except jelly). Spread
in 15 × 10 oblong pan lined with paper greased on both sides; bake 40
minutes. Remove from oven and run knife around edge. Turn out
onto towel, remove paper carefully; roll up immediately and let stand
one minute. Unfold; cool. Spread cake with dietetic jelly, roll, and
dust with granulated sugar substitute.

EASY SPONGE CAKE

Exchanges per serving: 1 slice = 1 Bread, ½ Lean Meat
Calories per serving: 100   Yield: 8 slices

1 cup egg whites (5–6)	1 cup flour
4 egg yolks	1 teaspoon baking powder
Non-nutritive sweetener	½ teaspoon vanilla *or*
equivalent to 1 cup	½ teaspoon lemon juice
sugar	

Preheat oven to 300°F. Beat egg whites very stiff; beat yolks until very light. Add half the sweetener to whites, the rest to yolks. Mix together and beat hard. Sift flour with baking powder; fold into egg mixture. Add vanilla or lemon juice. Pour into angel cake pan; bake 40 minutes, or until tester inserted in center comes out clean.

FRUIT SPONGE CAKE

Exchanges per serving: 1 serving = 1 Bread, ½ Lean Meat
Calories per serving: 84   Yield: 12 servings

1 tablespoon fresh orange	2 tablespoons fresh lemon
rind, grated	juice
½ cup fresh orange juice	½ teaspoon vanilla extract
4 eggs, separated	1½ cups flour
Non-nutritive sweetener	¼ teaspoon salt
equivalent to ½ cup	¾ teaspoon cream of tartar
sugar	

Preheat oven to 325°F. Combine rind and juice. Beat egg yolks until thick and lemon-colored, using highest speed of mixer. To juice and rind of orange, add sweetener, lemon juice, and vanilla extract. Sift flour and salt together; beat into egg yolks, alternating with liquid. Beat whites with cream of tartar until stiff peaks form. Fold the batter into the whites, being careful not to beat. Pour into 9″ ungreased tube pan; bake until done (about 1 hour). Invert pan on bottle to cool.

COFFEE SPONGE CAKE

Exchanges per serving: 1 serving = ½ Nonfat Milk
Calories per serving: 48 Yield: 10 servings

2 cups nonfat milk
2 tablespoons instant coffee
Non-nutritive sweetener
   equivalent to ¾ cup
   sugar

2 envelopes unflavored
   gelatin
6 egg whites

Scald nonfat milk. Dissolve coffee and ⅓ sugar substitute (equivalent to ¼ cup sugar) in scalded milk; chill until slightly thickened. Beat four egg whites stiff; fold in coffee mixture. Pour into mold; chill until firm. Beat remaining two egg whites, gradually adding remaining sugar substitute; continue beating until stiff. Spread over mold with spatula, bringing to edges.

POLLY'S DIETETIC JELLY ROLL

Exchanges per serving: 1 = ½ Bread, ½ Lean Meat
Calories per serving: 76 Yield: 12 servings

3 eggs, separated
Non-nutritive sweetener
   equivalent to ⅓ cup
   sugar
2 tablespoons orange juice
4 teaspoons liquid from
   any dietetic fruit
½ teaspoon lemon extract

1 cup flour
⅓ cup nonfat dry milk
1 teaspoon baking powder
¼ teaspoon salt
½ teaspoon cream of tartar
½ cup dietetic jelly

Preheat oven to 325°F. Mix egg yolks, sweetener, orange juice, liquid from fruit, and lemon extract. Beat 10 minutes with electric beater until very light and fluffy. Sift flour, dry milk, baking powder, and salt together three times. Very carefully fold sifted dry ingredients into whipped mixture. Beat egg whites and cream of tartar together until mixture stands in soft peaks. Fold into cake mixture. Pour into jelly-roll pan (about 15 × 10), which has been lined with lightly greased waxed paper. Bake about 20 minutes; cake will spring back when touched with finger. Remove from oven and run knife around edge. Turn out onto towel, remove paper carefully and roll up immediately; let stand one minute; unfold to cool. Fill with jelly and reroll. Slice to serve.

NOTE: Jelly roll must be kept in refrigerator. Any dietetic pudding mix may be used for filling. When pudding is set, beat and put in roll.

ORANGE CUPCAKES

Exchanges per serving: 1 cupcake = ½ Bread, ½ Fat
Calories per serving: 58   Yield: 30 cupcakes
(does not include frosting)

Non-nutritive sweetener equivalent to 1 cup sugar	¼ teaspoon salt
2 eggs, beaten	2 cups flour
⅔ cup orange juice, strained	2 teaspoons baking powder

Preheat oven to 325°F. Cream margarine and sweetener; add remaining ingredients. Beat one minute or longer in mixer at high speed. Pour into baking-cup-lined muffin tins. Bake until brown. Cool and frost, if desired.

CUPCAKES

Exchanges per serving: 1 cupcake = ¾ Bread, ½ Fat
Calories per serving: 107   Yield: 12 cupcakes

1½ cups flour	¼ teaspoon ground cloves
1½ teaspoons baking powder	½ cup diet margarine
½ teaspoon salt	2 eggs
¼ teaspoon baking soda	Non-nutritive sweetener equivalent to ⅔ cup sugar
½ teaspoon cinnamon	
½ teaspoon allspice	½ cup white raisins
½ teaspoon nutmeg	½ cup cold water

Preheat oven to 350°F. Combine flour, baking powder, salt, baking soda, cinnamon, allspice, nutmeg, and cloves; cut in margarine until size of small peas. Add remaining ingredients; mix until entire mixture is moistened. Place 12 paper baking cups in muffin tin and fill about half full; bake until tester inserted in center comes out clean.

GINGERBREAD

Exchanges per serving: 1 = 1 Bread, ½ Fat
Calories per serving: 73   Yield: 8 servings

4 tablespoons diet margarine

2 tablespoons molasses

½ teaspoon ginger

¼ teaspoon cinnamon

¼ teaspoon salt

1½ cups plus 1 tablespoon boiling water

1 cup rye flour

⅛ teaspoon baking powder

4 teaspoons baking soda

Preheat oven to 400°F. Measure margarine, molasses, ginger, cinnamon, and salt into bowl; add boiling water. Sift flour, baking powder, and baking soda into mixture; beat. Pour into greased oblong pan (15 × 10); bake 30 minutes.

CAKE FILLING

Exchanges per serving: 1 tablespoon = None
Calories per serving: 11   Yield: 1½ cups

1 recipe Lemon Frosting (see following recipe)

1 cup low-fat cottage cheese, drained and sieved

1½ teaspoons unflavored gelatin

2 tablespoons water

To Lemon Frosting, add cottage cheese; beat until smooth. Add gelatin to water and dissolve over boiling water (about 5 minutes). Blend carefully and use at once.

LEMON FROSTING

Exchanges per serving: 1 tablespoon = None
Calories per serving: 7   Yield: ⅓ cup

2 tablespoons nonfat dry
  milk
1½ tablespoons lemon juice
Non-nutritive sweetener
  equivalent to 2 table-
  spoons sugar

1 teaspoon vanilla
½ teaspoon unflavored
  gelatin
2 tablespoons water

Combine all ingredients except gelatin and water. Dissolve ½ teaspoon gelatin in 2 tablespoons water over hot water. Beat remaining ingredients at high speed of electric mixer about 15 minutes. Add gelatin gradually. Continue beating until frosting stands in peaks. Use immediately.

LOW-CALORIE FROSTING

Exchanges per serving: 1 tablespoon = ½ Fat
Calories per serving: 24   Yield: ¾ cup

4-ounce package
  Neufchâtel cheese
4 teaspoons nonfat milk

Non-nutritive sweetener
  equivalent to ½ cup
  powdered sugar
¼ teaspoon salt
1 teaspoon vanilla extract
Food coloring as desired

Cream cheese and nonfat milk thoroughly; add sweetener, salt, and vanilla; blend well. Add coloring last.
Note: If you wish to frost more than ½ dozen cupcakes, increase amounts accordingly.

CREAMY FROSTING

Exchanges per serving: 1 tablespoon = none
Calories per serving: 15   Yield: ½ cup

½ cup low-fat cottage
   cheese, sieved
⅛ teaspoon salt
½ tablespoon diet
   margarine, melted

Non-nutritive sweetener
   equivalent to ½ cup
   sugar
1 teaspoon almond or
   vanilla extract

Mix all ingredients; beat until smooth. Spread on cake. Frosts one 10″ cake.

COOKIES

BROWNIES DIVINE

Exchanges per serving: 1 brownie = ½ Bread, 1½ Fat
Calories per serving: 100   Yield: 16 brownies

½ cup diet margarine
Non-nutritive sweetener
  equivalent to 1¼ cups
  sugar
1 square unsweetened
  chocolate

1 teaspoon vanilla extract
2 eggs
¾ cup flour
1 teaspoon baking powder
½ cup nuts, chopped

Preheat oven to 350°F. Cream margarine and sweetener until light
and fluffy. Place chocolate in aluminum foil; melt over boiling water.
Stir chocolate into margarine mixture; beat until smooth. Beat in
vanilla and eggs. Sift and stir together flour and baking powder; add
nuts; stir this mixture into first mixture until smooth. Greast an 8"
square pan; pour in batter; bake until brownies are shiny, about 30
minutes. Cool in pan; cut into 16 pieces. Serve cool.

BROWNIES

Exchanges per serving: 1 brownie = ¼ Bread, 1 Fat
Calories per serving: 60   Yield: 48 brownies

1 cup diet margarine
2 squares unsweetened
  chocolate
2 cups flour
½ teaspoon salt
1 teaspoon baking soda

Non-nutritive sweetener
  equivalent to 2 cups
  sugar
4 eggs, well beaten
1 teaspoon vanilla extract
½ cup nuts, chopped

Preheat oven to 325°F. Melt margarine and chocolate over low heat;
set aside. Sift together flour, salt, and baking soda. Add sweetener,

eggs, and vanilla to margarine and chocolate; stir into dry ingredients until well blended; stir in nuts. Pour into 13 × 9 pan that has been sprayed well with pan coating. Bake 20 minutes; cool. Cut into 1½" squares.

TASTY DIET BROWNIES

Exchanges per serving: 1 brownie = ¼ Bread, 1 Fat
Calories per serving: 50   Yield: 16 brownies

⅔ cup flour, sifted
½ teaspoon baking powder
¼ teaspoon salt
1 ounce (1 square) unsweetened chocolate
1 egg

½ cup dietetic maple syrup
Non-nutritive sweetener
   equivalent to 2 tea-
   spoons sugar
⅓ cup walnuts, chopped
½ teaspoon vanilla extract

Preheat oven to 350°F. Measure flour; add baking powder and salt; sift again. Melt chocolate over hot water. Beat egg one minute; add maple syrup and sweetener; beat two more minutes. Add melted chocolate; blend. Add flour and stir (do not beat) until smooth. Add walnuts and vanilla. Spread batter ½" to ¾" thick in an 8" square pan or 9" pie tin. Bake 40 minutes.

CHOCOLATE BITES

Exchanges per serving: 1 cookie = ½ Fat, ¼ Bread
Calories per serving: 36   Yield: 2½ dozen cookies

⅓ cup diet margarine
¼ cup cocoa
¼ cup liquid artificial
   sweetener
2 eggs, well beaten

2 teaspoons vanilla extract
1 cup flour
½ teaspoon baking soda
½ teaspoon salt

Preheat oven to 325°F. Melt margarine; add cocoa, sweetener, eggs, and vanilla; stir until well blended. Sift flour, baking soda, and salt together; add and mix well (batter will be quite dry). Spread in well-greased 8" square pan. Bake about 20 minutes. Cool and cut into bites.

CHOCOLATE COOKIES

Exchanges per serving: 1 cookie, 2″ diameter = ¼ Bread
Calories per serving: 24   Yield: 2½ dozen cookies

1 egg, separated
Non-nutritive sweetener
    equivalent to ⅓ cup
    sugar
2 teaspoons unsweetened
    fruit liquid, any kind

1 cup flour
1 teaspoon baking powder
¼ teaspoon salt
½ cup dietetic chocolate
    topping
¼ teaspoon cream of tartar

Preheat oven to 325°F. Mix egg yolk, sweetener, and fruit liquid together in large bowl. Beat with electric mixer until light and fluffy (about 10–12 minutes). Meanwhile sift flour, baking powder, and salt together three times. Add chocolate topping to liquid mixture; beat until thoroughly mixed. Beat egg white with cream of tartar until it stands in soft peaks. Very carefully fold dry ingredients into chocolate topping mix. Fold beaten egg white into this mixture; drop by teaspoonfuls onto lightly greased cookie sheet. Bake about 10 minutes or until cookie springs back when lightly touched. Remove cookies with spatula to wire rack to cool.

MARY'S CHOCOLATE CHIP COOKIES

Exchanges per serving: 1 cookie = ¼ Bread, ½ Fat, without nuts
                                = 1 Fat, ¼ Bread, with nuts
Calories per serving: 40 without nuts   Yield: 3 dozen cookies
                      50 with nuts

¼ teaspoon salt
½ teaspoon baking soda
1 cup flour, sifted
½ cup diet margarine
Non-nutritive sweetener
    equivalent to ¾ cup
    sugar

½ teaspoon vanilla extract
1 egg, beaten
½ cup semisweet chocolate,
    shaved fine
½ cup nuts, if desired

Preheat oven to 375°F. Sift salt, baking soda, and flour together. Cream margarine; add sweetener, vanilla, and egg; blend well. Add flour mixture; beat well. Stir in chocolate; add nuts (if desired). Drop by level spoonfuls onto a lightly greased baking sheet. Bake about 10 minutes.

CRISP APPLESAUCE COOKIES

Exchanges per serving: 1 cookie = ¼ Bread, ¼ Fat, ¼ Fruit
Calories per serving: 35   Yield: 4 dozen ccookies

1⅔ cups flour, sifted
1 teaspoon cinnamon
¼ teaspoon nutmeg
¼ teaspoon cloves
½ teaspoon allspice
½ teaspoon salt
1 teaspoon baking soda
½ cup diet margarine

Non-nutritive sweetener
    equivalent to 1 cup
    sugar
1 egg
1 cup unsweetened apple-
    sauce
⅓ cup white raisins
1 cup whole bran cereal

Preheat oven to 375°F. Sift first 7 ingredients together. Beat margarine, sweetener, and egg until light and fluffy. Add flour mixture and applesauce alternately; mix well after each addition. Fold in raisins and cereal. Drop by teaspoonfuls onto well-greased sheet of heavy-duty aluminum foil, about 1" apart. Bake until golden brown (about 15 minutes).

REFRIGERATED COCONUT COOKIES

Exchanges per serving: 1 cookie = ¼ Bread, ¼ Fat
Calories per serving: 22   Yield: 2½ dozen cookies,
                                                         ¼" thick each

Non-nutritive sweetener
    equivalent to ½ cup
    sugar
¼ cup unsweetened fruit
    juice
1 teaspoon vanilla extract

¼ teaspoon baking powder
¼ teaspoon salt
1 cup flour
¼ cup diet margarine
2 tablespoons coconut

Preheat oven to 400°F. Combine sweetener, juice, and vanilla extract. Sift together baking powder, salt, and flour; cut in margarine.

Add liquid ingredients. After these are well mixed, work in coconut. Form dough into a roll about 7½" long, 2" in diameter; wrap in waxed paper and place in refrigerator until well chilled and firm. Slice into thirty ¼" thick cookies; place on ungreased cookie sheet. Bake 10 minutes.

COCONUT FRUIT COOKIES

Exchanges per serving: 1 cookie = ½ Bread, ¼ Fat
Calories per serving: 35   Yield: 3 dozen cookies

1½ cups flour
1 teaspoon baking powder
¼ teaspoon baking soda
¼ teaspoon salt
⅓ cup diet margarine
⅓ cup flaked coconut
1 egg

½ cup unsweetened fruit
  juice
2 teaspoons orange *or*
  lemon peel, grated
Non-nutritive sweetener
  equivalent to ⅓ cup
  sugar
1 teaspoon almond *or*
  vanilla extract

Preheat oven to 400°F. Combine flour, baking powder, baking soda, and salt; cut in margarine until consistency of peas. Stir in coconut; add remaining ingredients all at once. Stir with fork until dough holds together. Drop about 2" apart by teaspoonfuls onto an ungreased cookie sheet. Bake until light golden brown (about 10 minutes).

FRUIT COOKIES

Exchanges per serving: 1 cookie = ⅓ Bread, ½ Fat, ¼ Fruit
Calories per serving: 60   Yield: 20 cookies

½ cup flour
⅛ teaspoon cloves
¼ teaspoon nutmeg
1 teaspoon cinnamon
¼ teaspoon salt
½ teaspoon baking soda
½ cup raisins

½ cup rolled oats, uncooked
½ cup dietetic cranberry
  sauce
½ cup diet margarine,
  melted
1 egg
1 teaspoon vanilla extract

Preheat oven to 375°F. Sift flour, cloves, nutmeg, cinnamon, salt, and baking soda together; add raisins and oats. Combine cranberry sauce, margarine, egg, and vanilla extract. Stir into dry ingredients until they are moistened. Drop by teaspoonfuls onto lightly greased cookie sheet; bake 10–12 minutes.

SPICY APPLESAUCE COOKIES

Exchanges per serving: 2″ diameter cookie = 1 Bread, 1 Fruit
Calories per serving: 20   Yield: 3½ dozen cookies

1 cup flour
⅓ cup nonfat dry milk
1 teaspoon baking powder
½ teaspoon cinnamon
¼ teaspoon nutmeg
¼ teaspoon cloves
⅛ teaspoon salt
2 eggs

Non-nutritive sweetener
    equivalent to 8 tea-
    spoons sugar
3 tablespoons unsweetened
    fruit liquid (any fruit)
½ cup unsweetened apple-
    sauce
10 almonds blanched and
    cut in quarters

Preheat oven to 325°F. Sift dry ingredients together three times. Mix eggs, sweetener, and fruit liquid. Beat at top speed of mixer until fluffy and thick (about 10 minutes). Decrease speed; add applesauce and beat 3 minutes. Carefully fold in dry ingredients. Drop by teaspoonfuls onto lightly greased cookie sheet. Place ¼ almond on each cookie. Bake about 10 minutes. Cookie will spring back at light touch when done. (These may be placed under broiler to give deeper finish.)

ORANGE COOKIES WITH NUTS

Exchanges per serving: 1 cookie = ¼ Bread, ½ Fat
Calories per serving: 43   Yield: 2½ dozen cookies

½ cup frozen unsweetened   1 cup flour
   orange juice concentrate   ¼ teaspoon salt
1 egg   ¼ teaspoon baking powder
¼ cup diet margarine   1 teaspoon vanilla extract
Non-nutritive sweetener   ½ cup pecans, chopped fine
   equivalent to 1 cup sugar

Preheat oven to 375°F. Cream first four ingredients; beat well. Sift flour, salt, and baking powder; add to creamed mixture. Mix gently until just blended; add vanilla and nuts. Drop by teaspoonfuls onto lightly greased heavy-duty aluminum foil; bake until lightly browned (about 15 minutes).

ORANGE OR LEMON PEEL COOKIES

Exchanges per serving: 2 cookies = ½ Bread, 1 Fat
Calories per serving: 84   Yield: 4 dozen cookies

½ cup diet margarine   2 cups flour
Non-nutritive sweetener   1 teaspoon baking powder
   equivalent to ½ cup   ½ teaspoon salt
   sugar   ¾ cup pecans, chopped fine
⅓ cup hot water   1 tablespoon orange or
1 teaspoon orange extract   lemon peel, finely grated
1 teaspoon vanilla extract

Preheat oven to 400°F. Cream first five ingredients; sift together and add flour, baking powder, and salt. Blend in pecans and orange or lemon peel until mixture is smooth. Shape dough into roll about 2″ × 4″. Wrap in waxed paper; chill well in refrigerator. Cut roll into 48 cookies; place on lightly greased heavy-duty aluminum foil. Bake until brown around edges, about 12–15 minutes.

YUMMY PEANUT BUTTER COOKIES

Exchanges per serving: 1 cookie = ¼ Bread, ½ Fat, ¼ Lean Meat
Calories per serving: 45   Yield: 18 cookies

⅓ cup flour
¼ teaspoon baking soda
¼ teaspoon baking powder
¼ cup diet margarine
4 tablespoons peanut butter

Non-nutritive sweetener
  equivalent to 1 table-
  spoon brown sugar
Non-nutritive sweetner
  equivalent to ½ cup
  sugar
1 egg, well beaten

Preheat oven to 375°F. Grease cookie sheet lightly. Sift flour, baking soda, and baking powder. Work margarine and peanut butter with spoon until creamy; gradually add brown sugar substitute, continue working until light. Add regular sugar substitute and egg; beat well. Mix in dry ingredients thoroughly. Drop by teaspoonfuls onto lightly greased heavy-duty aluminum foil; flatten with tines of fork. Bake until done (about 8–10 minutes).

PEANUT BUTTER COOKIES

Exchanges per serving: 1 cookie = ½ Bread, 1 Fat
Calories per serving: 80   Yield: 8 cookies

8 graham cracker squares,
  crushed
2 tablespoons peanut butter
Non-nutritive sweetener
  equivalent to ¼ cup
  sugar

1 teaspoon baking powder
3 egg yolks
1 teaspoon nonfat milk

Preheat oven to 350°F. Combine graham cracker crumbs and peanut butter; add sweetener and baking powder. Add egg yolks and milk; mix well. Divide into eight 1″ cookies and press with tines of fork to flatten. Bake 10 minutes.

JOAN'S PEANUT BUTTER COOKIES

Exchanges per serving: 5 cookies = ½ Bread, 1½ Fat, ½ Lean Meat
Calories per serving: 116   Yield: 4 dozen cookies

¼ cup diet margarine	1 egg
Non-nutritive sweetener	⅓ cup nonfat milk
equivalent to 1 cup	1 teaspoon vanilla extract
sugar	1 cup flour
½ cup peanut butter,	¼ teaspoon salt
softened*	1 teaspoon baking powder

Preheat oven to 375°F. Combine margarine, sweetener and peanut butter and blend well. Combine egg, nonfat milk, and vanilla; add to first mixture. Sift flour, salt, and baking powder together; add, blending well. Drop by spoonfuls onto greased cookie sheet (or heavy-duty aluminum foil). Flatten with tines of fork dipped in water. Bake 10 minutes.

ANGEL'S KISS

Exchanges per serving: 1 kiss = ¼ Fat, ¼ Lean Meat
Calories per serving: 26   Yield: 3 dozen kisses

Non-nutritive sweetener	½ cup blanched almonds,
equivalent to 1½ cups	finely cut
confectioner's sugar	1 teaspoon instant diet
1½ cups egg	tea mix
yolks, beaten	1 teaspoon almond extract

Preheat oven to 325°F. Beat sweetener into yolks; add almonds, tea mix, and almond extract. Line muffin pans with paper baking cups; fill each half full. Bake until golden brown; remove cups while warm. Cool on wire rack.

*Leave at room temperature until sufficiently soft.

BUTTERMILK OAT COOKIES

Exchanges per serving: 1 square = ¼ Bread, ¼ Fat
Calories per serving: 29   Yield: 2½ dozen cookies

1 cup flour
¼ teaspoon baking soda
½ teaspoon salt
½ cup rolled oats, uncooked

Non-nutritive sweetener
    equivalent to 3 table-
    spoons sugar
¼ cup buttermilk
¼ cup diet margarine,
    melted

Preheat oven to 400°F. Sift flour, baking soda, and salt; add oats. Add sweetener to buttermilk; stir with margarine into flour mixture until dry ingredients are moistened. Knead dough lightly on well-floured board for a few minutes; roll thin. Cut into 2″ squares. Bake on ungreased cookie sheet until brown (10–12 minutes).

GRANDMA'S COOKIES

Exchanges per serving: 1 cookie = ½ Bread, 1 Fat
Calories per serving: 65   Yield: 2 dozen cookies

⅔ cup diet margarine
Non-nutritive sweetener
    equivalent to ¾ cup
    sugar
1 teaspoon vanilla extract
1 egg

4 teaspoons nonfat milk
2 cups all-purpose flour,
    sifted
1½ teaspoons baking
    powder
¼ teaspoon salt

Preheat oven to 375°F. Thoroughly cream margarine, sweetener, and vanilla. Add egg; beat until light and fluffy; stir in milk. Sift flour, baking powder, and salt together; blend into creamed mixture. Divide dough in half; chill 1 hour. Roll half of the dough at a time. (Keep balance chilled for easier rolling.) On lightly floured surface, roll dough to about ½″ thickness. Cut in desired shapes; bake 6–8 minutes. Cool slightly, remove from pan. Top each with unsweetened fruit, if desired. (See Fruit Exchange List for additional calorie count.)

BUTTERSCOTCH SQUARES

Exchanges per serving: 1 square = ½ Fat
Calories per serving: 25   Yield: 70 squares

½ cup diet margarine
Non-nutritive sweetner
  equivalent to 2 cups
  brown sugar
2 eggs

1½ cups flour
2 teaspoons baking powder
1 teaspoon vanilla extract
½ cup walnuts, chopped

Preheat oven to 350°F. Cook margarine and sweetener together until smooth. Cool to lukewarm. Add eggs; beat well. Add flour, baking powder, vanilla, and walnuts. Spread in lightly greased 13 × 9 pan. Bake 30 minutes. Cut into 1¼" squares. Sprinkle with non-nutritive granulated sugar substitute. Cool.

CREAM CHEESE DELIGHT

Exchanges per serving: 1 cookie = ¼ Bread, ½ Fat
Calories per serving: 58   Yield: 36 cookies

½ cup diet margarine
3 ounces Neufchâtel
  cheese
Non-nutritive sweetener
  equivalent to ⅓ cup
  sugar
1 egg yolk

1 teaspoon orange extract
1 teaspoon orange rind,
  grated
1 teaspoon lemon rind,
  grated
1½ cups flour, sifted
½ teaspoon salt

Preheat oven to 400°F. Cream softened margarine and cream cheese; add sugar substitute gradually and continue to cream until light and fluffy. Add egg yolk, extract, and rinds; beat well. Add flour and salt, which have been sifted together, to creamed mixture, a little at a time. Chill about 1 hour. Form into small balls; flatten with back of fork tines on ungreased cookie sheet. Bake until brown (10–12 minutes).

MACAROONS

Exchanges per serving: 1 macaroon = ½ Fat
Calories per serving: 24   Yield: 3½ dozen macaroons

1 egg, separated
Non-nutritive sweetener
  equivalent to 1 cup sugar
2 cups cornflakes

1 cup shredded coconut
½ cup chopped pecans
  (optional)
½ teaspoon almond extract

Preheat oven to 350°F. Beat egg white stiff but not dry; fold in sweetener. Add cornflakes, coconut, chopped pecans, and almond extract. Drop from teaspoon onto greased baking sheet; bake about 12 minutes. Remove at once from baking sheet.

SPICY COOKIES

Exchanges per serving: 1 cookie = ⅛ Bread, ½ Fat
Calories per serving: 30   Yield: 24 cookies

⅓ cup diet margarine
1 cup flour
¼ teaspoon baking powder
¼ teaspoon salt
2 tablespoons cocoa
1 tablespoon water

Non-nutritive sweetner
  equivalent to ⅓ cup
  sugar
½ teaspoon cinnamon
½ teaspoon nutmeg
1 teaspoon vanilla extract

Preheat oven to 375°F. Cream margarine until light and nearly cream-colored. Sift flour, baking powder, salt, and cocoa together; blend into margarine until smooth. Mix water, sweetener, cinnamon, nutmeg, and vanilla extract; add to flour-margarine mixture; mix until smooth (dough will be stiff). Shape into balls about ¾" round. Place on cookie sheet; flatten with blade of knife dipped in cold water. Bake until done (about 15 minutes). Remove from tray and cool.

MARY'S THUMBPRINTS

Exchanges per serving: 1 cookie = ¼ Fat, ¼ Bread
Calories per serving: 28   Yield: 4 dozen cookies
plus diet jelly (2 teaspoons = 16 calories)

½ cup diet margarine	½ teaspoon vanilla extract
Non-nutritive sweetener equivalent to ¼ cup sugar	1 tablespoon lemon juice
	1 tablespoon orange juice
1 tablespoon orange rind, grated	1 cup flour
	1 teaspoon salt
1½ teaspoons lemon rind, grated	1 egg, separated
	½ cup nuts, finely chopped
	Diet jelly

Preheat oven to 350°F. Mix together all ingredients except egg whites and nuts. Roll into small balls. Beat egg white stiff. Spread the nuts out on a piece of waxed paper. Roll each ball in egg white, then in nuts. Place on cookie sheet and make a thumbprint in each. Bake 12 minutes; cool. When cool, fill each thumbprint with diet jelly.

OATMEAL COOKIES

Exchanges per serving: 1 cookie = ¼ Bread, ⅓ Fat, ¼ Fruit
Calories per serving: 42   Yield: 4 dozen cookies

1½ cups quick-cooking or instant oatmeal, uncooked	1½ cups flour, sifted
	1 teaspoon baking powder
	½ teaspoon salt
⅔ cup diet margarine, melted	½ cup nonfat milk
	1 teaspoon vanilla extract
2 eggs, beaten	¼ cup raisins
Non-nutritive sweetener equivalent to 1½ cups sugar	

Preheat oven to 400°F. Measure oatmeal into bowl; stir in melted margarine; mix well. Stir in eggs and sweetener; add mixture of flour, baking powder, and salt alternately with the combined milk and vanilla. Add raisins. Drop onto cookie sheet from level teaspoon; bake until golden brown (about 10–15 minutes).

RICE FLOUR COOKIES

Exchanges per serving: 1 cookie = ¾ Bread, ¾ Fat
Calories per serving: 78   Yield: 2 dozen cookies

¾ cup diet margarine
Non-nutritive sweetener
  equivalent to 1½ cups
  sugar
2 eggs
½ teaspoon vanilla extract

½ teaspoon almond extract
1 teaspoon orange *or* lemon
  extract
2½ cups rice flour
1 teaspoon cream of tartar
1 teaspoon baking soda

Preheat oven to 375°F. Cream margarine and sweetener; add eggs and extracts. Sift flour, cream of tartar, and baking soda; mix all ingredients well; roll into small balls. Place on greased cookie sheet (or heavy-duty aluminum foil); flatten with tines of fork. Bake until brown (10 minutes).

PIES AND PIE CRUSTS

APPLE PIE

Exchanges per serving: 1 filling = 1 Fruit, ½ Fat
1 pastry = 2 Bread, ½ Fat
Calories per serving: filling, 75   Yield: 8 servings
pastry, 220

Non-nutritive sweetener
  equivalent to ¾ cup
  sugar
2 tablespoons flour
½ teaspoon cinnamon
Dash of nutmeg

Dash of salt
3 cups tart apples, pared,
  cored, and thinly sliced
Pastry for two-crust 9″ pie
2 tablespoons diet
  margarine

Preheat oven to 400°F. Combine sweetener, flour, spices, and salt; mix with apples. Line pie plate with pastry; fill with apple mixture; dot with margarine. Place top crust on pie; sprinkle with sugar substitute, if desired. Bake about 50 minutes, or until done.

DEEP-DISH APPLE PIE

Exchanges per serving: 1 serving = 1 Bread, 1 Fat, ½ Fruit
Calories per serving: 125   Yield: 8 servings

4 apples, pared and sliced
  thin
2 teaspoons lemon juice
½ teaspoon lemon rind,
  grated
¼ teaspoon nutmeg
½ teaspoon cinnamon

Non-nutritive sweetener
  equivalent to 1 cup
  sugar
½ tablespoon arrowroot
1⅛ teaspoons salt
1 cup flour, sifted
⅓ cup diet margarine
⅓ cup water

Preheat oven to 425°F. Combine apples, lemon juice, lemon rind, nutmeg, cinnamon, sweetener, arrowroot, and ⅛ teaspoon salt. Pour into well-buttered 9″ deep-dish pie plate. Combine flour and 1 teaspoon salt; cut in margarine until consistency of cornmeal; blend in water; roll out as for a pie crust; place on top of filling. Bake until crust is brown (about 35 minutes).

MYRA'S APPLE PIE

Exchanges per serving: 1 serving = 1 Bread, 2 Fat, 1 Fruit
Calories per serving: 200   Yield: 12 servings

2 cups flour	3 tablespoons lemon juice
Non-nutritive sweetener	1 cup water
equivalent to 1⅓ cup	10 apples, peeled, cored,
sugar	and sliced
¾ cup diet margarine	½ cup white raisins
1 egg	1 teaspoon cinnamon

Preheat oven to 375°F. Mix flour with about ⅔ of the sweetener; crumble margarine into flour mixture with fingers until mixture is size of peas. Stir in egg with fork until well blended. Work dough with hands until a smooth ball; divide into 3 sections. Wrap ⅓ dough in waxed paper; store in refrigerator until ready for top crust. Grease a 10″ springform pan lightly; press remaining ⅔ dough firmly and evenly over bottom and about ¾ up the sides of pan; set aside. Mix lemon juice and water; add apples a few at a time to the lemon-water to moisten each slice thoroughly. When apples are moistened, squeeze moisture out with hands and place apples in large bowl. Add raisins, balance of sweetener, and cinnamon. Stir and mix. Place in crust. Roll refrigerated ⅓ dough on well-floured board, to 1″ larger than pan. Fit dough over apples, pressing side and top together with wet fingers (so surface is flush with top). Prick pastry with fork several times; bake 1 hour and 10 minutes. Cool 10 minutes; loosen but leave in pan until room temperature.

GREAT APPLE AND GRAPE PIE

Exchanges per serving: 1 filling = ½ Fat, 2 Fruit
                      1 pastry = 1 Bread, 1 Fat
Calories per serving: filling, 100   Yield: 6 servings
                      pastry, 110

3 tablespoons tapioca
Dash of salt
3 cups apples, cored, pared,
   and sliced
2 cups seedless grapes, cut
   in halves
Pastry for one 9″ pie crust,
   unbaked

½ cup water
Non-nutritive sweetener
   equivalent to 1 cup
   sugar
2 tablespoons lemon juice
1 tablespoon diet margarine,
   melted

Preheat oven to 425°F. Mix tapioca and salt; toss with apples and grapes. Place in unbaked pie shell. Combine remaining ingredients; pour over fruit. Cover top with alumninum foil; bake 15 minutes. Reduce heat to 325°F. and continue baking until apples are tender (about 50 minutes).

QUICK APPLE PIE

Exchanges per serving: 1 filling = 1 Fruit
                      1 pastry = 2 Bread, 2 Fat
Calories per serving: filling, 40   Yield: 8 servings
                      pastry, 220

4 cups apples, pared, cored,
   sliced very thin
2 teaspoons lemon juice
¼ teaspoon lemon peel,
   finely grated
¼ teaspoon nutmeg

½ teaspoon cinnamon
1 tablespoon arrowroot
Non-nutritive sweetener
   equivalent to ¾ cup
   sugar
One recipe Rich Flaky
   Crust (see Index)

Preheat oven to 425°F. Mix together all ingredients except pastry. Prepare crust, lining an 8″ pie plate. Fill with apple mixture and top with second crust; flute edges. Make four or five cuts for air vents.

Lightly cover fluted edges with aluminum foil to prevent excessive browning of crust. After about 30 minutes, remove foil and continue baking until apples are tender (another 10–20 minutes). Cool.

SHERRY'S APPLE PIE

Exchanges per serving: 1 filling = 1 Fruit
                       1 pastry = 2 Bread, 2 Fat
Calories per serving: filling, 40   Yield: 6 servings
                   pastry, 220

5 apples, sliced   Dash of cinnamon
2 teaspoons tapioca   Pastry for two-crust 9″ pie
Non-nutritive sweetener
    equivalent to ½ cup
    sugar

Preheat oven to 400°F. Roll ½ crust recipe to fit a 9″ pie pan; arrange apple slices in crust; sprinkle tapioca, sweetener, and cinnamon over top. Roll out remaining crust; crimp edges securely over top (moisten edges between crusts with water if necessary); perforate in about six places. Bake until apples are tender (about 30 minutes).
NOTE: If a one-crust pie is desired, adjust exchanges per serving to 1 Bread, 1 Fat, and subtract 110 calories per serving.

JIFFY BANANA CREAM PIE

Exchanges per serving: 1 filling = 1 Fruit, ½ Nonfat Milk
                       1 pastry = 1 Bread, 1 Fat
Calories per serving: filling, 80   Yield: 8 servings
                   pastry, 115

2 packages dietetic vanilla   2 bananas, sliced (or other
    pudding mix   fruit, such as peaches,
2 cups nonfat milk   strawberries)
                             8″ baked pie crust

Prepare pudding mix, using nonfat milk; cool slightly. Cover bottom of pie shell with banana slices. Fill with pudding and let stand until set.

BERRY PIE

Exchanges per serving: 1 filling = ½ Fruit
                    1 pastry = 1 Bread, 1 Fat
Calories per serving: filling, 20   Yield: 8 servings
                    pastry, 110

1 quart berries (e.g., blue-berries, raspberries)	1 tablespoon arrowroot
2 teaspoons lemon juice	Non-nutritive sweetener equivalent to ¾ cup sugar
¼ teaspoon lemon peel, finely grated	Pastry for one 9″ pie crust, unbaked
½ teaspoon cinnamon	

Preheat oven to 425°F. Wash berries; mix with next five ingredients. Put into pie crust; bake until tender (45 to 50 minutes). If a two-crust pie is desired, cover pie before baking, cut vents in the top crust, flute edges, and cover fluting with aluminum foil to prevent excessive browning.

NOTE: For a two-crust pie, adjust exchanges per serving to 2 Bread, 2 Fat, and add an additional 110 calories.

BANANA CREAM PIE

Exchanges per serving: 1 filling = ⅓ Bread, ½ Nonfat Milk
                    1 pastry = 1 Bread, 1 Fat
Calories per serving: filling, 75   Yield: 6 servings
                    pastry, 110

Pastry for one 9″ pie crust	Non-nutritive sweetener equivalent to ½ cup sugar
¼ cup flour	⅛ teaspoon salt
1½ cups nonfat milk	1 medium banana
1 egg, beaten	Nondairy whipped topping (optional) (10–15 calories per tablespoon)
1 teaspoon lemon juice	
½ teaspoon vanilla extract	

Bake and cool pie shell. Blend flour with ½ cup cold nonfat milk. Scald remaining 1 cup nonfat milk; add flour-milk mixture and egg, lemon juice, vanilla, sweetener, and salt. Cook in top of double boiler, stirring until thick. Slice banana into pie shell. Spread cream filling over top; cool. Cover with nondairy whipped topping, if desired. Use immediately.

CHIFFON EGGNOG PIE

Exchanges per serving: 1 filling = ½ Fat, ⅓ Nonfat Milk
                                    1 pastry = 1 Bread, 1 Fat
Calories per serving: filling, 57   Yield: 6 servings
                                    pastry, 110

1 envelope unflavored gelatin	¼ teaspoon salt
¼ cup cold water	½ tablespoon arrowroot
1½ cups nonfat milk	2 eggs, separated
Non-nutritive sweetener equivalent to ¾ cup sugar	1 teaspoon almond extract
	1 tablespoon rum extract
	9″ baked pie crust

Soften gelatin in cold water. Combine ¾ cup nonfat milk, sweetener, and salt in top of double boiler. Make a paste of arrowroot and remaining milk; stir into first mixture. Cook over boiling water, stirring constantly until thick. Beat egg yolks and add a little of the hot mixture; stir into remaining hot liquid in double boiler. Cook another 2 minutes; remove from heat; stir in softened gelatin until dissolved. Chill until mixture begins to set; stir in extracts. Beat egg whites very stiff; fold into gelatin mixture. Pour into baked pie shell; chill until firm. If desired top with Low-Calorie Topping Whip (see Index) or artificial whipped cream; sprinkle chocolate shavings over this.

NOTE: Add additional calories and exchanges if Low-Calorie Topping Whip is used.

ICEBOX CHOCOLATE PIE

Exchanges per serving: 1 serving = ½ Bread, ⅓ Fat, ¼ Nonfat Milk
Calories per serving: 97   Yield: 8 servings

2 tablespoons cocoa
⅛ teaspoon salt
1½ teaspoons arrowroot
½ cup nonfat milk, scalded
1 egg, separated

Non-nutritive sweetener
  equivalent to ¾ cup
  sugar
½ cup evaporated milk,
  beaten
1 teaspoon vanilla
12 graham cracker squares

Mix cocoa, salt, and arrowroot; blend in nonfat milk. Add slightly beaten egg yolk and sweetener; cook in top of double boiler until thickened; cool. Beat egg white, evaporated milk, and vanilla until stiff; fold into first mixture. Roll graham crackers into crumbs; sprinkle half in 8″ pie pan; pour in filling. Sprinkle remaining crumbs on top. Put in freezer until firm.

PEACHY PIE

Exchanges per serving: 1 serving = ½ Bread, 2 Fruit
Calories per serving: 110   Yield: 6 servings

1½ cups cornflakes
1 tablespoon diet mar-
  garine, melted
1 teaspoon hot water
4 cups unsweetened canned,
  or fresh peaches, sliced*
2 envelopes dietetic cherry
  gelatin

1 tablespoon lemon juice
1 teaspoon lemon rind,
  grated
¼ cup nonfat dry milk
¼ cup cold water
Non-nutritive sweetener
  equivalent to 3 table-
  spoons sugar

Preheat oven to 325°F. Crush cornflakes. Mix margarine and hot water; add to cornflakes; mix thoroughly. Spread mixture evenly in an 8″ pie pan; press firmly around edge with spatula. Bake 8–10 minutes; cool. Drain peaches, reserving juice; add water to make 1

*If using fresh peaches use 1 cup water in lieu of juice.

cup liquid. Dissolve gelatin in liquid. Heat almost to boiling; add 2 tablespoons lemon juice and rind; cool. Chop and add peaches; chill until mixture begins to thicken. Mix nonfat dry milk, cold water, and remaining lemon juice; whip until mixture stands in peaks. Add sweetener; beat until mixture stands in very stiff peaks. Very carefully fold gelatin-peach mixture into whipped milk; mix. Pour gently into pie shell; serve chilled.

PEACH PIE

Exchanges per serving: 1 filling = ½ Fruit
                  1 pastry = 1 Bread, 1½ Fat
Calories per serving: filling, 26   Yield: 10 servings
               pastry, 125

2 cups firm, ripe peaches
¼ tablespoon salt
Water
Non-nutritive sweetener
   equivalent to ½ cup
   sugar
¼ teaspoon lemon juice
Pastry for one 10″ pie crust,
   unbaked
2 tablespoons diet mar-
   garine

Preheat oven to 325°F. Peel and pit peaches; slice and drop into solution of salt and 1 quart hot water; drain. Mix sweetener, ¼ cup water, and lemon juice together; pour over peaches. Set in refrigerator until cool. Place in unbaked 10″ pie crust; dot with margarine. Bake until peaches are tender to the touch of a fork (30–40 minutes).

PEACH COBBLER

Exchanges per serving: 1 serving = ¾ Bread, ½ Fruit
Calories per serving: 78 per ⅛ cobbler   Yield: 8 servings

4 fresh peaches, peeled and
   cut into ⅛″ slices
1 tablespoon lemon juice
1 teaspoon lemon rind,
   finely grated
1 tablespoon arrowroot
1 tablespoon allspice
¼ teaspoon salt
Non-nutritive sweetener
   equivalent to ½ cup
   sugar
½ cup flour
3 tablespoons diet mar-
   garine

Preheat oven to 425°F. Spray pie plate with Pam or other nonfat spray. Combine fruit, juice and lemon rind in large mixing bowl. Combine arrowroot, allspice, ½ the salt, and the sweetener; mix well. Place over peaches and shake bowl gently to coat all pieces of fruit; spread peaches evenly in pie plate. Make crumb mixture of flour, remaining salt, and diet margarine; spread evenly over top of peaches. Bake until crumbs are nicely browned, 35–40 minutes. Serve hot.

CHIFFON PUMPKIN PIE

Exchanges per serving: 1 filling = ½ Lean Meat, ¼ Nonfat Milk,
                                    ½ Bread
                         1 pastry = 1 Bread, 1 Fat
Calories per serving: filling, 93   Yield: 8 servings
                      pastry, 110

Pastry for one 9″ pie crust	½ teaspoon salt
1 envelope unflavored gelatin	4 eggs, separated
1 cup evaporated milk	Non-nutritive sweetener equivalent to ¾ cup sugar
½ cup water	
½ teaspoon nutmeg	1¼ cups canned pumpkin, mashed
½ teaspoon cinnamon	
¼ teaspoon ginger	

Line a 9″ pie plate with desired crust. Bake and cool. Combine next eight ingredients, reserving egg whites; beat well. Stir and cook in top of double boiler until consistency of medium white sauce (about 10 minutes). Stir in sweetener. Place in refrigerator until cold. Beat whites until they form soft peaks. Fold pumpkin into gelatin mixture; add beaten egg whites carefully; pour into pie shell and chill until set.

OLGA'S PUMPKIN PIE

Exchanges per serving: 1 serving = 1½ Bread
Calories per serving: 110   Yield: 6 servings

1½ cups cornflakes
1 teaspoon diet margarine,
   melted
1 tablespoon hot water
½ cup dietetic maple syrup
1 cup nonfat milk

2 envelopes dietetic butter-
   scotch or vanilla pudding
1 cup pumpkin, canned or
   fresh cooked
1 egg

Preheat oven to 325°F. Crush cornflakes. Mix margarine and water;
add to cornflakes; mix thoroughly. Spread mixture evenly in a 9″ pie
pan; press firmly around edge with spatula. Bake 8–10 minutes; cool.
Blend remaining ingredients in saucepan; cook over medium heat,
stirring constantly until mixture comes to a boil. Cool to room
temperature; pour into pie shell. Chill at least three hours before
serving.

PUMPKIN PIE

Exchanges per serving: 1 serving = ¼ Lean Meat, ¾ Milk, 1/6 Bread
Calories per serving: filling, 135   Yield: 8 servings
                      pastry, 110

1½ cups canned or fresh
   cooked pumpkin
Non-nutritive sweetener
   equivalent to ¾ cup
   sugar
½ teaspoon salt
1¼ teaspoons cinnamon
½ to 1 teaspoon ginger

¼ to ½ teaspoon nutmeg
¼ to ½ teaspoon cloves
2 eggs, slightly beaten
1¼ cups nonfat milk
2 cups nonfat evaporated
   milk
Pastry for one 9″ pie crust,
   unbaked

Preheat oven to 400°F. Combine pumpkin, sweetener, salt, and
spices thoroughly; blend in eggs, milk, and evaporated milk. Pour
into unbaked pastry shell; bake until knife inserted between center
and outside comes out clean. Serve cool.

MARY C'S PUMPKIN PIE

Exchanges per serving: 1 filling = ¼ Nonfat Milk, ½ Bread
1 pastry = 1 Bread, 1 Fat
Calories per serving: filling, 90   Yield: 6 servings
pastry, 110

1 egg	½ teaspoon ginger
Non-nutritive sweetener equivalent to 1 cup sugar	¼ teaspoon cloves
	1½ cups canned pumpkin
¾ teaspoon allspice	¾ cup evaporated milk
¾ teaspoon nutmeg	¾ cup fresh orange juice
¾ teaspoon cinnamon	One 9″ pie crust, unbaked

Preheat oven to 425°F. Combine egg, sweetener, spices, and pumpkin; blend well. Add milk and orange juice gradually; stir until well blended. Pour into unbaked pie shell; bake 10–12 minutes, then reduce heat to 325°F.; bake until a knife inserted near center comes out clean (about 45 minutes).

POLLY'S PUMPKIN PIE

Exchanges per serving: 1 filling = ¼ Lean Meat, ½ Nonfat Milk, 1½ Bread
1 pastry = 1 Bread, 1 Fat
Calories per serving: filling, 120   Yield: 8 servings
pastry, 110

Non-nutritive sweetener equivalent to 1 cup sugar	½ teaspoon cloves
	1¾ cups evaporated milk
1½ teaspoons cinnamon	2 eggs, well beaten
½ teaspoon allspice	1½ cups canned pumpkin
½ teaspoon ginger	One 9″ unbaked pie shell, chilled
½ teaspoon nutmeg	

Preheat oven to 425°F. Combine sweetener and spices; stir in evaporated milk and eggs; add pumpkin. Beat until smooth. Pour mixture into a chilled 9″ pie shell (do not prick bottom of shell). Bake at

425°F. for 15 minutes, then reduce heat to 350°F.; bake until knife inserted in center of pie comes out clean (about 35–40 minutes). Cool.

FRUIT FILLING FOR PIE

Exchanges per serving: 1 filling = 1 Fruit
1 pastry = 1 Bread, 1 Fat
Calories per serving: filling, 40   Yield: 8 servings
pastry, 110

4 cups any fruit (apples, blueberries, fresh peaches, pears, orange sections, pineapple, seedless grapes, etc.)
Non-nutritive sweetener equivalent to ¾ cup sugar

1 tablespoon arrowroot
¼ teaspoon lemon peel, grated fine
2 teaspoons lemon juice
¼ teaspoon nutmeg
½ teaspoon cinnamon
Pastry for one 9″ pie crust, unbaked

Preheat oven to 425°F. Mix all ingredients together and place in pie crust. Bake until fruit is tender (about 45–50 minutes). If a two-crust pie is desired, cover unbaked pie with second crust, cut air vents in top, and flute edges. Cover fluted edges with foil to prevent excessive browning (remove foil after 30 minutes), and bake as before.
NOTE: For a two-crust pie, adjust exchanges per serving to 2 Bread, 2 Fat, and crust calories to 220.

RICE CEREAL PIE CRUST

Exchanges per serving: 1 serving = ¼ Fat, ⅛ Bread
Calories per serving: 26   Yield: One 8″ crust

1 cup crispy rice cereal, crushed
2 tablespoons diet margarine, melted

Non-nutritive sweetener equivalent to 4 tablespoons sugar

Mix ingredients together; line bottom and sides of 8″ pan; chill well before adding any desired filling.

FRUIT COBBLER

Exchanges per serving: 1 serving = 1 Bread, 1½ Fruit, ¼ Lean Meat
Calories per serving: 150   Yield: 4 servings

2 cups water-packed fruit
  (*e.g.*, cherries), un-
  sweetened; reserve juice
¼ teaspoon lemon juice
⅛ teaspoon almond extract
½ teaspoon arrowroot
⅔ cup juice from fruit
½ cup flour, sifted

⅛ teaspoon salt
¾ teaspoon baking powder
1 tablespoon diet margarine
1 egg
2 tablespoons nonfat milk
Non-nutritive sweetener
  equivalent to ¼ cup
  sugar

Preheat oven to 425°F. Place a layer of drained fruit in a shallow cake pan. Combine lemon juice, almond extract, arrowroot, and drained fruit juice; pour over fruit. Mix flour, salt, and baking powder; cut in margarine until mixture is like coarse sugar. Mix egg, nonfat milk, and sweetener; stir into dry ingredients; spoon onto fruit. Bake until browned (25–30 minutes). Serve warm.

MARGARET'S GLAZED BERRY TARTS

Exchanges per serving: 1 filling = ¾ Fruit
                       1 pastry = 1 Bread, 1½ Fat
Calories per serving: filling, 40   Yield: 6 servings
                      pastry, 143

Pastry for 6 medium tarts
1 envelope unflavored
  gelatin
¼ cup cold water
4 cups fresh berries, hulled
  and washed (*e.g.*, strawberries, boysenberries)

Non-nutritive sweetener
  equivalent to 1½ cups
  sugar
3 drops food coloring
2 tablespoons lemon juice

Preheat oven to 425°F. Bake tart shells until lightly browned. Remove from oven; let cool. Soften gelatin in cold water. Sweeten berries with sweetener and press through strainer until 1½ cups are obtained. Add coloring and lemon juice; bring to a boil; remove from heat. Add softened gelatin; stir to dissolve. Chill until mixture begins to thicken. Arrange remaining whole berries in baked shells. Cover with gelatin-berry mixture. May be topped with artificial cream or Low-Calorie Topping Whip (see Index).

YUMMY FRUIT TARTS

Exchanges per serving: 1 filling = 1 Fat, 1 Fruit
 1 pastry = 1 Fat, ½ Bread
Calories per serving: filling, 100   Yield: 6 tarts
 pastry, 115

1 tablespoon arrowroot
⅛ teaspoon salt
Non-nutritive sweetener equivalent to 1 cup sugar
1 cup fresh orange juice
1 cup unsweetened pineapple chunks

2 eggs, beaten
1 medium banana, sliced thin
¼ cup dried coconut, shredded
1 recipe Lorene's Graham Cracker Crust (see Index)

Combine arrowroot, salt, sweetener, and orange juice. Drain pineapple, reserving liquid; add sufficient water to make 1 cup. Combine liquid, arrowroot mixture, and beaten eggs. Cook over medium heat, stirring constantly, until mixture boils and thickens; remove from heat. Chill; fold in pineapple chunks, sliced banana, and coconut. Place in crust; chill until ready to serve.

CRUMBLY PIE CRUST

Exchanges per serving: 1 serving = ½ Fat
Calories per serving: 27   Yield: One 9″ crust

3 tablespoons diet margarine
Non-nutritive sweetener equivalent to 1 tablespoon sugar

¾ cup cornflake crumbs

Preheat oven to 375°F. Mix margarine, sweetener, and crumbs; press into 9″ pie plate with back of spoon. Press into bottom and up sides of plate (crust will be fairly thin).

RICH FLAKY CRUST

Exchanges per serving: ⅛ of single pie crust = 1 Bread, 1 Fat
Calories per serving: 125 (single crust)   Yield: two 8″ crusts

2 cups flour, sifted   ½ cup oil
1 teaspoon salt   3 tablespoons cold water

Preheat oven to 450°F. Sift flour and salt together; dribble oil on surface; stir with fork until completely mixed. Add cold water to form smooth ball. Divide dough in half. Place half on waxed paper; cover with another piece of waxed paper; roll dough to 12″ circle. Peel off paper; fit into pie plate. For one-crust pie, flute edges with moistened fork (or finger). Bake until browned (12–15 minutes); cool before filling. For two-crust pie, place one crust (unbaked) into pie plate, put in filling, and top with other crust. Slit upper crust in several places. Bake according to filling instructions. For two-crust pie, allow 2 Bread and 2 Fat exchanges, and adjust calories to 250 per serving.

PIE CRUST

Exchanges per serving: ⅛ crust = 1 Bread, 1½ Fat
Calories per serving: 130   Yield: one 8″ crust

1⅓ cups flour, sifted   ½ cup diet margarine,
½ teaspoon salt   melted
                                  2 tablespoons cold water

Sift flour and salt together; dribble margarine over surface. Stir with fork until completely mixed; add water to margarine-flour mixture; stir to smooth ball. Roll out dough to fit 8″ pie plate. Flute edges with fork. Refrigerate if crust is to be filled prior to baking. If baked unfilled, make several cuts with sharp knife in bottom and sides of crust. Bake at 450°F. until golden brown (13–15 minutes).

LORENE'S GRAHAM CRACKER CRUST

Exchanges per serving: 1 serving = 1 Bread, 1 Fat
Calories per serving: 115   Yield: one 9″ crust

1 cup (16) graham crackers,
  crushed fine
3 tablespoons diet mar-
  garine, melted

Non-nutritive sweetener
  equivalent to 2 table-
  spoons sugar

Preheat oven to 350°F. Combine ingredients well; press firmly into a
9″ pie plate. Bake about 10 minutes. Chill before filling.

PASTRY

Exchanges per serving: 1 serving = 1 Bread, 1 Fat
Calories per serving: 110   Yield: one 8″ crust

1 cup flour, sifted
1 teaspoon salt

5 tablespoons diet
  margarine
4 tablespoons water

Preheat oven to 425°F. Combine flour and salt; cut in margarine until
consistency of peas. Add water slowly until dough is moistened and
holds together. Knead dough lightly, pressing into a ball. Flour
pastry board and rolling pin; roll gently, turning often. Roll thin; lay
pastry over 8″ pie tin; press down gently, fluting edges. Slit bottom in
a few places with sharp knife. Bake until golden brown (about 14–15
minutes). Fill with desired filling. Use extra dough for individual
pastries.

CANNING AND FREEZING

CANNING FRUITS

To can fruits, use unsweetened fruit juice or water in place of the usual sugar syrup. Be sure to adhere to processing time and other instructions. When serving, count your fruit exchanges as you would for the commercially prepared sugar-free fruits.

Toss the fruit in lemon juice solution to keep it from darkening. Use sweetener equivalent to 2 to 4 cups of sugar for every 2 to 3 quarts of liquid; if this is not sweet enough (or too sweet), change to suit your taste. The U.S. Department of Agriculture, Washington, DC 20402, has some excellent books on canning that you may wish to send for before trying any recipes.

Use orange or pineapple juice, unsweetened, to obtain an unusual flavor. (These generally settle to the bottom of the jars, so shake well just before serving.) Raspberries and strawberries may be mashed and the juice saved; mixing this juice with water makes an excellent canning liquid.

Apples, grapes, peaches, pears, pineapple, and seedless oranges are fine to mix. A good variation is a half-and-half mixture of peaches and pears. Avoid fruits such as bananas, blueberries, cherries, plums, raspberries, and strawberries in fruit cocktail. (Bananas turn brown and become too soft, while the other fruits "weep" and become too liquid.)

Plums are fine for canning, but be sure you select the proper varieties. Use half water and half plum juice for the canning liquid to help keep the color from being lost.

FREEZING FRUITS WITHOUT SUGAR

Wash and drain thoroughly blackberries, blueberries, cranberries, currants, gooseberries, grapes, pineapple chunks, plums, raspberries, or rhubarb. Leave about ½ inch at top of container when packing. Freeze.

Figs, peaches, and strawberries go into special containers, covered with the ascorbic acid water solution (1 teaspoon crystalline ascorbic acid dissolved in each quart of water). Package, leaving 1 inch at top of quarts and ½ inch for pints. Freeze. Thaw frozen fruits until only a few ice crystals remain and sweeten as desired with non-nutritive sweetener.

VEGETABLES

Nearly any vegetable that can be cooked is recommended for freezing. Order the freezing booklet from the Department of Agriculture, Washington, DC 20402.

CUCUMBER PICKLES

Exchanges per serving: ½ cup = 1 Vegetable
Calories per serving: 25   Yield: 3 pints

6 cucumbers	¼ cup water
¼ cup salt	2 cups white vinegar
Non-nutritive sweetener equivalent to ¾ cup sugar	2 tablespoons pickling spice

Wash and dry cucumbers; cut into strips about 4″ long. Place in large bowl; sprinkle with salt. Let stand overnight. In the morning, rinse and drain well several times. Combine sweetener, water, and vinegar in large pan; bring to boil. Tie pickling spice in a cheesecloth bag and add to boiling ingredients. Add cucumbers; reduce heat; simmer about 15 minutes. Place cucumbers in clean hot pint jars. Heat liquid once more to boiling, pour over pickles in jars. Seal immediately.

ANNE'S CHILI SAUCE

Exchanges per serving: 1 tablespoon = 1 free Vegetable
Calories per serving: 6   Yield: 3 quarts

8 cups tomatoes, peeled
   and chopped
¼ cup red peppers,
   chopped fine
½ cup green peppers,
   chopped fine
1½ cups onion, chopped
   fine
1½ cups celery, chopped
   fine
Non-nutritive sweetener
   equivalent to ½ cup
   sugar

1 tablespoon salt
1½ cups cider vinegar
1 tablespoon Tabasco sauce
1 whole stick cinnamon
1 teaspoon cloves
1½ teaspoons celery seed
1½ teaspoons mustard seed
1 teaspoon Mei Yen
   seasoning

In a large heavy pan combine first nine ingredients. Combine spices
in a cheesecloth bag; add to first mixture. Bring to boil; reduce heat
and simmer. Stir occasionally, simmering for about 5–6 hours.
Remove bag of spices; pour remainder into clean, hot, pint jars; seal
immediately.

JAMS AND JELLIES

JAMS AND JELLIES WITHOUT SUGAR

Cover jars completely with water and bring water to boil. Boil 15 to 20 minutes. Remove jars from water (hold tongs under boiling water 60 to 90 seconds before removing jars so jars do not break); drain jars upside down on aluminum foil until just before using, then turn right side up.

Use your favorite non-nutritive sweetener, being careful to use the proper amount. Stir until it is completely dissolved and mixed. (Do not reboil.)

In top of double boiler, over low heat, melt the paraffin. Pour jam or jellies into jars carefully, and pour on melted paraffin to a thickness of about ¼ inch. Cool. Place in refrigerator. Keep refrigerated, and after first opening, be sure to keep covered with tight lid or aluminum foil molded to top.

APPLE BUTTER JELLY

Exchanges per serving: 1 tablespoon = ¼ Fruit
Calories per serving: 10   Yield: 5¾ cups

8 cups apples, cored, washed and cut in quarters	¼ teaspoon nutmeg
	1 teaspoon powdered cloves
2 cups unsweetened apple juice	¼ teaspoon anise seed, ground fine
¼ cup lemon juice	Non-nutritive sweetener equivalent to ½ cup sugar
¼ cup cider vinegar	
2 teaspoons lemon peel, ground fine	

Mix all ingredients except sweetener; bring to a boil, stirring constantly; boil a few minutes. Remove from heat, stir in sweetener. Ladle into jelly glasses and seal.

RUTH'S RASPBERRY JAM

Exchanges per serving: 1 tablespoon = trace Fruit
Calories per serving: 8   Yield: 2 cups

1½ teaspoons unflavored
  gelatin
1½ tablespoons cold water
3 cups fresh raspberries,
  crushed

Non-nutritive sweetener
  equivalent to ⅔ cup
  sugar
¼ teaspoon lemon juice
3 drops red food coloring
  (optional)

Soften gelatin in cold water. Combine berries and sweetener in saucepan; place on high heat; stir constantly until mixture boils. Remove from heat; add softened gelatin. Return to heat; cook for another minute. Remove and blend in lemon juice and food coloring. Place in pint jar; seal and store in refrigerator.

ANNE'S APPLE JELLY

Exchanges per serving: 1 tablespoon = ¼ Fruit
Calories per serving: 10   Yield: 2 cups

2 teaspoons unflavored
  gelatin
2 tablespoons lemon juice
⅛ teaspoon salt
1 teaspoon arrowroot

2 cups apple juice,
  unsweetened
Non-nutritive sweetener
  equivalent to 2 cups
  sugar

Mix gelatin, lemon juice, salt, and arrowroot. Stir in apple juice and boil, stirring constantly, for two minutes. Remove from heat; stir in sweetener. Fill jelly jars, seal, and store.

BLUEBERRY JAM

Exchanges per serving: 1 tablespoon = trace Fruit
Calories per serving: 6   Yield: 2½ cups

2 tablespoons lemon juice
3 teaspoons unflavored
  gelatin
⅛ teaspoon salt
1½ teaspoons arrowroot

2½ cups frozen unsweet-
  ened blueberries, par-
  tially thawed
Non-nutritive sweetener
  equivalent to 2 cups
  sugar

Mix lemon juice, gelatin, salt, and arrowroot; stir in blueberries. Boil gently until mixture thickens; stirring constantly (about 3–4 minutes). Stir constantly, boiling at full boil for 2 minutes. Remove from heat; stir in sweetener. Fill and seal jars.

PHYL'S APPLE JELLY

Exchanges per serving: 1 tablespoon = ¼ Fruit
Calories per serving: 10   Yield: 2 cups

4 teaspoons unflavored
  gelatin
2 cups unsweetened apple
  juice
Non-nutritive sweetener
  equivalent to 1 cup
  sugar

1½ teaspoons lemon juice
3 drops food coloring
  (yellow or green)

Soften gelatin in ¼ of the apple juice. Bring the remaining 1½ cups of juice to boil; remove from heat; add softened gelatin. Stir until gelatin dissolves; add sweetener, lemon juice, and food coloring. Bring to rolling boil. Place in clean pint jars; seal. Store in refrigerator.

APPLE-LEMON JELLY

Exchanges per serving: 1 tablespoon = ¼ Fruit
Calories per serving: 9   Yield: 2 cups

1 package unflavored
   gelatin
2 tablespoons lemon juice
⅛ teaspoon salt
1 teaspoon arrowroot

2 cups apple juice,
   unsweetened
Non-nutritive sweetener
   equivalent to 2 cups
   sugar

Mix gelatin, lemon juice, salt, and arrowroot; add apple juice and
boil, stirring constantly, for two minutes. Remove from heat; add
sweetener. Fill prepared jelly jars; seal.

STRAWBERRY JELLY

Exchanges per serving: 1 tablespoon = trace Fruit
Calories per serving: 5   Yield: 5½ cups

2 envelopes unflavored
   gelatin
½ cup lemon juice
Dash of salt
1 tablespoon arrowroot

4 cups strawberries, hulled,
   washed, and strained
Non-nutritive sweetener
   equivalent to 4 cups
   sugar

Mix gelatin, lemon juice, salt, and arrowroot; add strawberries. Boil,
stirring constantly, about 3 minutes. Remove from heat; stir in
sweetener. Fill and seal jars.

PINEAPPLE-APRICOT JAM

Exchanges per serving: 1 tablespoon = ⅓ Fruit
Calories per serving: 15   Yield: 5 cups

2 cups dried apricots
2 cups water
4 cups unsweetened pine-
   apple tidbits

2 tablespoons lemon juice
Dash of salt
Non-nutritive sweetener
   equivalent to 1 cup
   sugar

Boil apricots in water until tender (about 25 minutes). Drain pineapple tidbits and cut each one in half. Purée apricots and water with lemon juice and salt. Return to saucepan; stir in pineapple. Boil a few minutes, stirring now and then. Remove from heat; add sweetener. Fill jelly jars; seal.

CONSERVE

Exchanges per serving: 1 tablespoon = ½ Fat, ½ Fruit
Calories per serving: 42   Yield: 2 cups

1 cup dried apricots	2 tablespoons lemon juice
2 cups water	Non-nutritive sweetener
2¼ cups unsweetened pine-	equivalent to 1 cup
apple tidbits	sugar
⅛ teaspoon salt	½ cup nuts, finely chopped

Boil apricots in water until tender; purée. Drain pineapple tidbits; cut each piece into smaller pieces. Put apricot purée in saucepan; add pineapple, salt, and lemon juice. Boil slowly, stirring constantly, about 5 minutes. Remove from heat; stir in sweetener and nuts. Fill jars; seal.

JOAN'S CHUTNEY

Exchanges per serving: ¼ cup = 1 Fruit
Calories per serving: 45   Yield: 1½ pints

¾ cup white raisins	Non-nutritive sweetener
¼ cup bell peppers,	equivalent to 2 cups
chopped fine	sugar
1 cup white vinegar	½ teaspoon ginger
4 pears, cored, pared, and	¼ teaspoon allspice
chopped	¼ teaspoon cloves
	¼ teaspoon salt

Combine all ingredients in large pan; bring to boil. Reduce heat to medium; cook until pears are tender and mixture is slightly thick (about an hour). Spoon into three clear ½-pint jars and seal immediately.

CONVERTING THESE RECIPES FOR MICROWAVE OVENS

When you've found a recipe in our book you would like to use, try to find a similar one in your microwave recipe book. The amounts of ingredients in these recipes should match the ingredients in the microwave recipe. Make sure the dish is recommended for micro-cooking and is similar in size, shape, and cooking temperature.

Compare the corresponding cooking method and be sure you follow all directions carefully—including directions for covering the dish or not and whether waxed paper or Saran Wrap is to be used in any covering.

Refer to general information on food categories for each ingredient in your microwave cookbook. Also check the charts for meats and vegetables, suggested cooking times, and weights.

Certain types of food vary in cooking times: bread has very little moisture content, while vegetables have more moisture content and require longer times; potatoes and egg whites, which have little sugar or fat, take longer to cook than such foods as egg yolks and certain fruits, because the latter contain a greater amount of fat or sugar.

Be sure foods cooked in the microwave oven are not overcooked. Check them frequently. When you first try converting recipes, you will have to experiment. Allow for extra time to prepare these recipes.

Remember that the foods continue to cook once they are removed from the microwave oven, so remove them at the correct time. This is usually 10 to 20 minutes for meat and 5 to 10 minutes for vegetables.

It may be necessary to decrease the amount of liquid or increase the thickening agent in the diabetic recipes, as liquids evaporate more slowly in a microwave oven. You may also need to adjust the liquid if the recipe calls for short cooking time.

Lack of evaporation intensifies flavors, so it is generally best to add herbs, seasonings, and spices by taste after cooking, or else reduce amounts you'd usually use. Salt, in particular, should be added *last*, as it draws out moisture in the foods when microwaved. (Meat and vegetables should *not* be salted until cooking is finished.) Cloves, garlic, garlic powder, onion and other seasoning blends may be used in lieu of salt and will not have the drying effect of salt.

Because there is a lack of dry heat source, breads (quick and yeast), cakes, and cookies develop in a unique way—they are fluffier since they are not restricted by a crust. As steam rises to the surface after cooking, the tops of cakes will be moist and wet-looking. They will toughen if you overcook, as this removes the moist appearance from these baked goods. With the exception of chocolate, baked products will be pale and not crusty. We suggest using about ½ the amount of baking powder and soda when you are adapting one of our recipes for microwaving. To help prevent an irregular-shaped top, a lower power setting is preferable. It's best to use recipes for cookies that do not need browning and are soft, such as bars, etc. We do not suggest baking angel food and chiffon cakes in the microwave.

Following are some microwave conversion examples.

MEATLOAF

Regular recipe:
1 egg
2 cups ground beef (lean)
3 slices bread, cubed fine
¼ cup catsup (See Index)
⅓ cup onion, chopped fine

Conversion:
1 lb. lean ground beef
2 slices white bread (day old) cubed
3 tablespoons milk
2 tablespoons finely chopped onion
1 egg
2 tsp. Worcestershire Sauce
½ teaspoon salt
dash of pepper

Preheat oven to 400°F. Mix all ingredients well. Form into loaf. Place in 9 × 5 pan; bake until done (15–20 minutes).

Combine all ingredients. Spread in 9 × 5 ungreased glass or ceramic loaf dish. Microwave at High 17–21 minutes, or until center is firm and meat has lost its pink color, (internal temperature 145 to 150°F.). Rotate dish after half the cooking time. Let stand 5 to 10 minutes.

CRUMB CRUST

1 cup (16) graham crackers, crushed fine
3 tablespoons diet margarine, melted
Non-nutritive sweetener equivalent to 2 tablespoons sugar

Preheat oven to 350°F. Combine ingredients well; press firmly into a 9″ pie plate. Bake about 10 minutes. Chill before filling.

To adapt to microwaving without changing ingredients: Use graham crackers, chocolate or vanilla wafers, or ginger snaps. Melt margarine in 9″ glass or ceramic pie plate. Stir in crumbs and sweetener, if used. Press firmly against bottom and sides of plate using another pie plate or a ramekin to press evenly in pie plate. Microwave 1½ minutes, turning after 1 minute. Let cool before filling.

HINTS AND TIPS FOR MICROWAVING

Selecting Recipes for Conversion

It's best to start with a familiar recipe while you're learning conversion techniques. It helps to adapt it for microwaving when you know how the food is supposed to look and taste. Make sure the flavors and the proportions seem pleasing if you have not yet tried our recipe.

Then check the list of foods that won't work! (See your own microwave oven cookbook.) Can you achieve the cooking technique by microwaving?

Microwaving is a natural for moist cooking—check for recipes that call for covering, liquid, or steaming as this shows the food needs moisture and should do well in the microwave. It is much more satisfactory to use a conventional oven if a crust or dry surface is essential to the recipe.

Some foods may be slightly different when microwaved even though they can be adapted. Cakes will be more tender, omelets won't brown or have a crust—but you may even prefer the microwave version.

To help foods microwave evenly, stir or turn foods over. Recipes should adapt easily if our recipe allows for stirring or turning. Can you include stirring in a microwave recipe if ours does not call for stirring? Yes, rotate the dish and reduce the power setting if the recipe would be changed by too much stirring.

Select a recipe in your microwave cookbook with the same quality and quantity of main bulky ingredients, and a similar amount and type of liquid. (Liquid may be either like chicken broth, which you can microwave at "high," or delicate, like cream, which may take a lower power setting.)

Cubed sirloin is a higher quality meat that is microwaved in a different way than cubed chuck, as chuck is a less tender cut.

More food takes more time, so quantity is important. Follow the conversion guidelines; but if our recipe calls for a different amount of food you will need to adjust the cooking time.

Substituting Ingredients

You can generally make the same substitutions you ordinarily use for any of our recipes. For instance, if you prefer to use dried onions rather than fresh, follow directions on the package and use them in microwaving. Most seasonings are interchangeable—you can substitute any herb you like, in any recipe, for one you may not care for. Some substitutions—such as using process cheeses, which melt more smoothly, instead of dry or hard natural cheeses—are recommended for microwaving. "Quick-cooking" rice can be substituted for raw or converted rice; in the short time it takes to microwave the other ingredients in your casserole, the rice will be tender.

But you should be more careful with those substitutions that affect the microwaving times, method, or power setting.

You may need medium or a lower power, and double the time, if you substitute cream for milk. If using converted rice rather than quick-cooking rice, be sure to microwave the rice until partially tender before adding other ingredients. If flour is used in lieu of cornstarch in a sauce, increase amount as you would normally do and stir the sauce more frequently.

The consistency of a dish may be affected by some substitutions. If you are using yogurt rather than sour cream, reduce the amount because yogurt is more liquid.

Selecting the Microwave Method for One of Our Recipes

You can achieve most of the cooking methods called for in these recipes by microwaving.

Don't try deep-frying! This and boiling are the two conventional cooking methods that cannot be achieved with microwaving.

1. **TO OVEN BAKE:** Preheat oven and cook foods, covered or uncovered, at recommended temperature. If steam is desired, place a pan of water in oven.

   TO MICROWAVE BAKE: Using recommended power setting, microwave food, covered or uncovered. (Never preheat oven.)

2. **TO BRAISE, CASSEROLE, ROAST, STEW:** Sometimes fruit, meat, and vegetables are browned first, then simmered in liquid in a covered pan, generally on top of range or in oven. Stew takes more liquid than braising. Casseroles and roasted meats don't need additional liquid as they are cooked on a bed of moist vegetables.

   TO MICROWAVE BRAISE, CASSEROLE, ROAST, STEW: Do not brown; reduce amount of liquid. Use a cooking bag or cover tightly and microwave at "medium" or "medium low."

3. **TO PAN-BROIL OR PAN-FRY:** Cook food uncovered to keep crisp and dry. For pan-broiling do not use fat; use a small amount of fat for pan-frying.

   TO MICROWAVE PAN-BROIL OR PAN-FRY: Follow directions for preheating browning utensil. If broiling, add no fat; if pan-frying add fat. Microwave food, uncovered, on both sides.

4. **TO POACH:** Chicken, eggs, fish, and fruit are gently simmered in liquid to cover.

   TO MICROWAVE POACH: To produce steam, reduce liquid to 1 cup or less. Using plastic wrap, tightly cover dish. The type of food will determine power setting.

5. **TO ROAST:** Elevate meat on a rack placed in a shallow pan.

Cook uncovered to desired internal temperature, basting occasionally to keep surface moist.

TO MICROWAVE ROAST: Meat should be placed on a rack in uncovered baking dish. Turn meat over after half the cooking time, but it is not necessary to baste. Microwave at "medium" or "medium-low," using probe or microwave thermometer.

6. **TO SAUTÉ:** Brown or sear food in butter or oil. Cover and simmer over low heat. Add small amount of liquid or moist vegetables to chicken or meat.

TO MICROWAVE SAUTÉ: Unless desired for flavoring, omit fat and browning. Find the proper power setting suitable for the food and microwave, covered.

7. **TO STEAM:** Set a rack over boiling water and place food on it, or surround container of food with simmering water, in covered pot. Do not allow water to touch food in either case.

TO MICROWAVE STEAM: Microwave moist foods in a tightly covered dish. Do not use water. If cooking delicate foods, such as mousse, place the mold in a dish of hot water and microwave uncovered.

8. **TO STIR-FRY:** Using a small amount of oil, fry small pieces of food quickly. Stir constantly to prevent sticking. Add quick-cooking foods last; if desired, add sauce.

TO MICROWAVE STIR-FRY: Follow directions for preheating browning dish. Add oil and long-cooking foods. Stir every 2 minutes. Add quick-cooking foods last. If desired, add sauce.

Testing and Timing Microwave Recipes for Doneness

Cooking time is the major difference between these recipes and the microwave adaptation. Check your microwave oven for wattage. If yours has a very high wattage, check to see if your food is done *before* the minimum time. Varying speed and evenness of cooking are found in different microwave ovens. Some may be slower with heavy or light loads, and some operate more efficiently with a medium food load. The cookbook you received with your own microwave oven will help you in estimating minimum and/or maximum times. It is possible your book may recommend stirring or turning more frequently—good results may depend on the extra attention suggested.

Unless the food is one that needs more time to rehydrate or tenderize, generally the microwaving time will be approximately a fourth to a half of the conventional time. Don't believe that in microwaving a few seconds' difference can ruin the food. Cooking times help you *estimate* how long the food may take in both conventional and microwaving ovens, but *you* are the final judge of when it is done.

1. **ADD:** If you see it is needed to match consistency of our recipe, add a little more liquid.

2. **DON'T ADD:** Be sure you reduce salt and DO NOT add until recipe is done.

3. **SCALE:** To help estimate cooking time according to weight of food and power setting, a microwave scale is a very useful tool.

4. **STIR:** If food seems to be cooking unevenly, rotate the dish or turn the food.

5. **TASTE:** When cooking is completed, especially the first time you convert a recipe, taste! (This is also a big help in judging consistency, tenderness, and texture.)

6. **TEST:** Doneness tests are, for most recipes, the same for conventional ovens as for microwave ovens. Check for doneness at the minimum time; overcooking is a real problem, and you can always cook longer! Don't forget to allow for standing time when required.

7. **WATCH:** Frequently check the progress of cooking. It does not harm the food to interrupt the cooking.

CONVECTION OVENS

Makers say that cooking in shorter periods and at lower temperatures are the advantages to the convection ovens. The fan blows hot air around foods and the air circulation cooks on all exposed sides.

These are not as good as regular ovens in every category of food, for quality, in our opinion, but you can use any recipe in our book in one of the convection ovens. Be sure you watch the food so it is not cooked too rapidly. You must experiment with any new oven and this is no exception!

HOW TO USE NUTRITION LABELING TO WORK OUT FOOD EXCHANGES

Many foods are now labeled with carbohydrate, fat, and protein information. We felt the following material would be most helpful.

This method was developed by the Diabetes Education Center, Minneapolis, MN, and is made available through the cooperation and courtesy of The Pillsbury Company and in particular Ms. Suzanne J. Carlson, Pillsbury Department of Nutrition.

FOOD EXCHANGES USING NUTRITION LABELING

This method uses the Exchange List for Meal Planning developed by the American Diabetes Association, Inc., and the American Dietetic Association, and is offered here through the courtesy of The Pillsbury Company. Should you have questions about using the following Exchange List, consult your dietition or physician.

Many food products now carry nutrition labeling on the package. This nutrition information makes it possible for diabetics to include many more foods in their diets, using the method that is described here.

```
           One 10″ Cheese Pizza
        Nutrition Information
            per Serving
   Serving size  . . . . . . .½ pizza
   Servings per container . . . . .2
   Calories per serving  . . . .438
   Protein . . . . . . . . . .22 grams
   Carbohydrates  . . . . .52 grams
   Fat  . . . . . . . . . . . . .16 grams
```

Any company that uses nutrition labeling must follow the format set out by the FDA. This is the part of the information you need to work out the exchanges.

How to Work Out Food Exchanges

You need this exchange list for reference:

Exchange	Calories*	Carbo-hydrate	Protein	Fat
1 Milk (non-fat) Exchange	80	12 grams	8 grams	trace
1 Vegetable Exchange	25	5 grams	2 grams	—
1 Fruit Exchange	40	10 grams	—	—
1 Bread (starch) Exchange	70	15 grams	2 grams	—
1 Meat Exchange, Lean	55	—	7 grams	3 grams
Medium Fat	78	—	7 grams	5.5 grams
High Fat	100	—	7 grams	8 grams
1 Fat Exchange	45	—	—	5 grams

We will use the pizza label shown before as an example. With practice, this method can be used for other food products with nutrition labeling and used for various serving size of a product. You need this information from the nutrition label:

Serving size . . . . ½ pizza
Servings per container 2
Calories per serving 438
Protein . . . . 22 grams
Carbohydrates . . . . . 52 grams
Fat . . . . 16 grams

	Exchanges	Carbohydrate	Protein	Fat
1. List the grams of carbohydrate, protein, and fat from pizza label		52	22	16
2. Divide the carbohydrate (52 gm) by 15 gm to get the number of Bread Exchanges ($52 \div 15 = 3^7/_{15}$, which is rounded to 3 Bread Exchanges*)	Bread—3			
List the carbohydrate, protein, and fat in the 3 Bread Exchanges.		−45	− 6	0
Subtract from label values		7	16	16
3. Divide the remaining carbohydrate (7) by 5 gm to get the number of Vegetable Exchanges.**	Veg.—1			
List the carbohydrate, protein, and fat values for the Vegetable Exchange.		− 5	− 2	0
Subtract from label values.		2	14	16
4. Divide the remaining protein (14) by 7 gm to get the number of Meat Exchanges.	Med. Fat Meat—2			
List the carbohydrate, protein, and fat values for Meat Exchanges.		0	−14	−11
Subtract from label values		2	0	5
5. Divide the remaining fat (5) by 5 gm to get the Fat Exchange.	Fat—1	0	0	−5
List and subtract.		2	0	0

	Exchanges	Carbo-hydrate	Protein	Fat
6. Therefore, one serving of pizza is equivalent to 3 Bread, 1 Vegetable, 2 Medium-Fat Meat and 1 Fat Exchanges.				
7. As a final check, ½ pizza	52 gm	22 gm	16 gm	428
Exchanges (3 Bread, 1 Vegetable, 2 Meat, and 1 Fat)	50 gm	22 gm	16 gm	436

*Carbohydrate and protein provide 4 calories/gm; fat provides 9 calories/gm.
**Count whole and nearest ½ exchanges; disregard less.

DIABETIC EXCHANGES FOR PACKAGED FOODS

	Serving size	Milk	Vege-table	Bread	Lean Meat	Fat	Calories
SOUP MIXES (prepared)							
Lipton Cup-a-Soup							
Bean soup mix	6 oz.			1	½		106
Vegetable-beef soup mix	6 oz.		1				25
Cream-style chicken soup mix	6 oz.			⅔		1	91
Cream of mushroom soup mix	6 oz.			⅔		1	91
Beef-flavored noodle soup mix	6 oz.			½			35
Chicken noodle with meat soup mix	6 oz.			½			35
Green pea soup mix	6 oz.			1½	½		157
Cream of tomato soup mix	6 oz.			1		½	141
Spring vegetable soup mix	6 oz.		2				50

	Serving size	Milk	Food Exchanges Vege-table	Bread	Lean Meat	Fat	Calories
Nestlé Souptime							
Chicken noodle soup mix	6 oz.			½			35
Beef noodle soup mix	6 oz.			½			35
Cream of chicken soup mix	6 oz.			⅔		1	91
Tomato soup mix	6 oz.			1			70
French onion soup mix	6 oz.		1				25
Green pea soup mix	6 oz.			1	½		106
Mushroom soup mix	6 oz.			⅔		1	91
Cream of vegetable soup mix	6 oz.		1½			r	82
BREADS AND CRACKERS (prepared)							
Pillsbury							
Refrigerated Hot Loaf	1 slice			1		½	93
Refrigerated apple-cinnamon muffins	1 muffin			1		1	115
Refrigerated corn muffins	1 muffin			1½		1	150
Refrigerated plain buttermilk biscuits	2 biscuits			1½			105

	Serving size	Food Exchanges					Calories
		Milk	Vege-table	Bread	Lean Meat	Fat	
Refrigerated butterflake dinner rolls	1 roll			1		½	93
Refrigerated crescent rolls	1 roll			1		1	115
Applesauce bread mix, 16 slices per loaf	1 slice			1½		½	128
Apricot-nut bread mix, 16 slices per loaf	1 slice			1½		½	128
Banana bread mix, 16 slices per loaf	1 slice			1½		½	128
Blueberry-nut bread mix, 16 slices per loaf	1 slice			1½		½	128
Cherry-nut bread mix, 16 slices per loaf	1 slice			1½		1	150
Cranberry bread mix, 16 slices per loaf	1 slice			1½		½	128
Date bread mix, 16 slices per loaf	1 slice			1½		½	128
Nut bread mix, 16 slices per loaf	1 slice			1½		½	128
Oatmeal-raisin bread mix, 16 slices per loaf	1 slice			1½		½	128
Hot roll mix	1 roll			1		½	93

	Serving size	Milk	Vege-table	Bread	Lean Meat	Fat	Calories
Nabisco							
Animal crackers	4 crackers			½		¼	47
Oyster crackers	12 crackers			½		¼	47
Plain chocolate wafers	3 wafers			1		½	93
Graham crackers	2 crackers			¾		¼	64
Thin pretzel sticks	34 sticks			½			35
Arrowroot biscuits	4 biscuits			1		½	93
Plain vanilla wafers	5 wafers			1		½	93
Saltine crackers	7 crackers			1		½	93
Shredded wheat wafers	5 wafers			1		½	93
Thin wheat crackers	13 crackers			1		1	105
Zwieback toast	3 pieces			1		½	93
DESSERTS (prepared)							
General Foods							
Fruit-flavored gelatin	½ cup			1			70
Cheesecake mix	⅛ of 8" cake			2½		2	265

Food Exchanges

	Serving size	Food Exchanges					Calories
		Milk	Vege-table	Bread	Lean Meat	Fat	
Egg custard mix (prepared with milk)	½ cup	½		1		1	160
Low-calorie pudding (prepared with nonfat milk)	½ cup	½		½			75
Pillsbury							
Apple, blueberry, or cherry turnovers	1 turnover			1½		1½	173
Brownie mix	2 1½" squares			1		1	105
Gingerbread mix	3" square			2		1	185

MAIN DISHES

Kraft

	Serving size	Food Exchanges					Calories
		Milk	Vege-table	Bread	Lean Meat	Fat	
Macaroni & cheese dinner mix	¾ cup			2	½	2½	280
American-style spaghetti dinner mix	1 cup			3		1	255

	Serving size	Milk	Vegetable	Bread	Lean Meat	Fat	Calories
Cheese pizza mix	¼ box			2½	1	1	275
Sausage pizza mix	¼ box			2½	1	1½	298
Betty Crocker							
Chili-tomato Hamburger Helper mix	1/5 pkg.			2		½	163
Hamburger stew Hamburger Helper mix	1/5 pkg.			1½			105
Lasagna Hamburger Helper mix	1/5 pkg.			2			140
Spaghetti Hamburger Helper mix	1/5 pkg.			2			140
Cheeseburger macaroni Hamburger Helper mix	1/5 pkg.			2		1	195
Creamy Noodles 'n Tuna or Hamburger Helper Mix	1/5 pkg.			2		2	230
Creamy Rice 'n Tuna or Hamburger Helper Mix	1/5 pkg.			2		1	195
Mrs. Paul's							
Frozen deviled crab cakes	1 cake			1	1 high-fat	1	170
Frozen fish sticks	4 sticks			1	1 high-fat	½	148

Food Exchanges

MEAL ACCOMPANIMENTS

	Serving size	Milk	Food Exchanges Vege- table	Bread	Lean Meat	Fat	Calories
Ore-Ida							
Frozen French fries	3 oz.			1½		1	150
Frozen cottage fries	3 oz.			1½		1½	173
Frozen Southern-style hash brown potatoes	3 oz.			1			70
Frozen shredded hash brown potatoes	3 oz.			1½		2	70
Frozen plain Tater Tots	3 oz.			1½		2	195
Frozen onion rings	2½ oz.			1		2	160
Van Camps							
Canned Spanish rice	1 cup			2		1	185
Betty Crocker							
Instant mashed potato buds (dry)	⅓ cup			1			70
Dry scalloped potato mix	⅛ pkg.			1½			105
Dry hash brown potato mix	⅛ pkg.			1½			105

| | Serving size | Milk | Food Exchanges | | | | |
			Vege-table	Bread	Lean Meat	Fat	Calories
Green Giant							
Frozen broccoli in cheese sauce	3½ oz.		1		½		85
Frozen cauliflower in cheese sauce	3½ oz.		1			1	85
Frozen creamed peas	3½ oz.			1		1	115
Minute							
Packaged precooked rice mixes (beef-flavored, Spanish, chicken-flavored, fried)	½ cup			2		1	185
Stove Top							
Packaged stuffing mix (prepared with butter)	½ cup			1½		2	195
Birdseye							
Frozen French-style green beans with mushrooms	3.5 oz.		1		½		53

	Serving size	Milk	Food Exchanges Vege- table	Bread	Lean Meat	Fat	Calories
Frozen corn and peas with to- matoes	3.3 oz.			1			70
Frozen mixed vegetables with onion sauce	2.6 oz.		2			1	95
Frozen green peas and onions	3.3 oz.		2				50
Frozen rice and peas with mush- rooms	2.3 oz.			1½			105
Frozen Bavarian-style beans with spaetzle	3.3 oz.		2				50
Frozen Chinese-style vegetables	3.3 oz.		1				25
Frozen Danish-style vegetables	3.3 oz.		1				25
Frozen Italian-style vegetables	3.3 oz.			½			35
Frozen Japanese-style vegetables	3.3 oz.		1				25
Frozen Mexican-style vegetables	3.3 oz.			1			70

Betty Crocker

	Serving size	Milk	Vege- table	Bread	Lean Meat	Fat	Calories
Packaged noodles almondine mix (prepared)	¼ pkg.			2		2	230
Packaged noodles Romanoff mix (prepared)	¼ pkg.	½		1		2	320

SAUCE MIXES

Durkee

	Serving size	Milk	Vege-table	Bread	Lean Meat	Fat	Calories
				Food Exchanges			
Spaghetti sauce mix (made with tomato paste)	¼ pkg.			1			70
Hollandaise sauce mix	¼ pkg.			⅓		½	46
Cheese sauce mix	¼ pkg.			⅓		½ med.-fat	101
Sour cream sauce mix (made with whole milk)	¼ pkg.			⅓		½	46
Teriyaki sauce mix	¼ pkg.			¼			18
Taco seasoning mix	¼ pkg.			¼			18
Brown gravy mix	¼ pkg.			¼			18
Chicken gravy mix	¼ pkg.			⅓			18

	Serving size	Milk	Food Exchanges Vege-table	Bread	Lean Meat	Fat	Calories
MISCELLANEOUS							
Pet							
Canned imitation sour cream	1 tbsp.					½	23
Dry nondairy coffee creamer	1 tbsp.					½	23
Contadina or Hunts							
Canned pizza sauce	1 cup			1½		1	150
Canned tomato sauce	1 cup			1			70
Seasoned bread crumbs	3 tbsp.			1			70
Canned tomato paste	¾ cup			2			140

RECOMMENDATIONS FOR USING OTHER BRAND-NAME PRODUCTS IN EXCHANGE LISTS

	Serving size ½ can (prepared ounces)	Milk	Vege-table	Bread	Lean Meat	Fat	Calories
			Food Exchanges				

CAMPBELL

Condensed Soups

	Serving size ½ can (prepared ounces)	Milk	Vege-table	Bread	Lean Meat	Fat	Calories
Asparagus, cream of	10			1		1	100
Bean with bacon	11			2	1	½	200
Beef	11			1	1		110
Beef broth (bouillon)	10		1				35
Beef noodle	10			1			90
Black bean	11			1½			150
Celery, cream of	10			½		1½	110
Cheddar cheese	11	1				3	200
Chicken alphabet	10			1		1	110
Chicken broth	10				1		50
Chicken, cream of	10			½		2	140

	Serving size ½-can (prepared ounces)	Food Exchanges					Calories
		Milk	Vege-table	Bread	Lean Meat	Fat	
Chicken 'n dumplings	10			½	1	1	120
Chicken gumbo	10			1	1		70
Chicken noodle	10			1			90
Chicken NoodleO's	10			1			90
Chicken with rice	10			1			80
Chicken and Stars	10			1			80
Chicken vegetable	10			1			90
Chili beef	11			2	1	½	210
Clam chowder (Manhattan)	10			1		½	100
Clam chowder (N.Eng. made with whole milk)	10	½		1	1	1	200
Consommé (beef)	10				1		45
Curly noodle with chicken	10			1		½	100
Golden vegetable NoodleO's	10			1			90
Green pea	11			2	1		190
Hot dog bean	11			2	1	1	230
Meatball alphabet	10			1	1	½	140
Minestrone	10			1		½	110

	Serving size ½ can (prepared ounces)	Food Exchanges						Calories
		Milk	Vegetable	Bread	Lean Meat	Fat		
Mushroom, cream of	10			1		2		150
Mushroom, golden	10			1		1		110
Noodles & ground beef	10			1		1		110
Onion	10			1				80
Onion, cream of (made with water & whole milk)	10	½		1		1½		180
Oyster stew (made with whole milk)	10	½		½		2		170
Pepper pot	10			1	1	½		130
Potato, cream of (made with whole milk)	10	½		1		1		140
Scotch broth	10			1		1		100
Shrimp, cream of (made with whole milk)	10	½		1		2		210
Split pea with ham & bacon	11			2	1	½		230
Stockpot	11			1	1			130
Tomato			1	1				110
Tomato (made with whole milk)	10	½	1	1		1½		210
Tomato-beef NoodleO's	10			1½		1		160

	Serving size ½ can (prepared ounces)	Food Exchanges					Calories
		Milk	Vege-table	Bread	Lean Meat	Fat	
Tomato bisque	11			2		½	160
Tomato rice, old-fashioned	11			2		½	160
Turkey noodle	10			1			80
Turkey vegetable	10			1			90
Vegetable	10		1	1			100
Vegetable beef	10			½	1		90
Vegetable, old fashioned	10			1			90
Vegetarian vegetable	10			1			90

Soup for One

	1 can (prepared ounces)	Milk	Vege-table	Bread	Lean Meat	Fat	Calories
Bean, old fashioned	11⅜			2		1	210
Clam chowder, N.Eng. (made with whole milk)	11⅜	½		1		1	200
Golden chicken & noodles	11⅜			1	1	1	120
Mushroom, cream of, with wine	11¼			1		2	160
Tomato royale	11⅜			2		1	180
Vegetable, old world	11⅜			1		1	125

| | Serving size ½ can (prepared ounces) | Food Exchanges | | | | | | Calories |
		Milk	Vege-table	Bread	Lean Meat	Fat	
Chunky Soups	½ can (undiluted ounces)						
Chunky beef	9½			1	2		190
Chunky chicken	9½		1	1	2		200
Chunky chicken with rice	9½			1	2		160
Chunky chicken vegetable	9½			1½	1	1	190
Chunky chili beef	9½			2	2		260
Chunky clam chowder (Manhattan)	9½			1½	1		160
Chunky minestrone	9½			1½	1		160
Chunky old fashioned bean with ham	9½		1	2	1	1	260
Chunky old fashioned vegetable beef	9½		1	1	1		160
Chunky sirloin burger	9½		1	1	1	1	210
Chunky split pea with ham	9½			1	2		220
Chunky steak & potato	9½			1	2		190
Chunky turkey	9½		1	1	1		160
Chunky vegetable	9½		1	1		1	140

	Serving size ½ can (prepared ounces)	Food Exchanges						Calories
		Milk	Vege-table	Bread	Lean Meat	Fat		
Low Sodium Products	1 can (ounces)							
Chunky beef, low sodium	7½		1	1	1	1		170
Chunky chicken, low sodium	7½		1	1	1	1		170
Green pea, low sodium	7¼		1	1	1			150
Mushroom, cream of, low sodium	7¼			½		2		140
Tomato, low sodium	7¼		1	1		1		130
Turkey noodle, low sodium	7¼			1				60
Vegetable, low sodium	7¼			1				90
Vegetable beef, low sodium	7¼		1		1			80
"V-8" cocktail vegetable juice, low sodium	6		1					35
Chili con carne with beans, low sodium	7¾			2	2	1½		310

| | Serving size ½ can (prepared ounces) | Food Exchanges | | | | | Calories |
		Milk	Vege-table	Bread	Lean Meat	Fat	
GENERAL FOODS							
Potatoes (one portion prepared as directed)							
AuGratin				1½		1	150
Creamed				1½		1	160
Sour cream 'n chive				1		1	140
Scalloped				1½		1	150
Hash browns with onions				1½		1	150
Julienne				1		1	130
Potato Buds				1		1	130
Mug-o-Lunch (one pouch or one portion)							
Spaghetti and tomato sauce				2½			160
Macaroni and cheese sauce		½		2		1	230
Noodles and beef flavored sauce				2		½	170

	Serving size ½ can (prepared ounces)	Milk	Vege-table	Bread	Lean Meat	Fat	Calories
				Food Exchanges			
Chicken flavored noodles and sauce				2		½	150
Oriental noodles and sauce				2		½	190
Hamburger Helper (one portion prepared as directed)							
Hamburger stew			1	1		1	290
Hash dinner				1½	2 med. fat	1	300
Chili tomato			1	1½	2 med. fat	½	320
Lasagne				2	2 med. fat	½	330
Hamburger pizza dish				2	2 med. fat	½	340
Potato stroganoff				2	2 med. fat	½	330

	Serving size ½ can (prepared ounces)	Milk	Vege-table	Bread	Lean Meat	Fat	Calories
			Food Exchanges				
Rice oriental	8 oz. pkg.			2	2 med. fat	½	340
Rice oriental	6½ oz. pkg.			1½	2 med. fat	½	300
Spaghetti				2	2 med. fat	½	330
Beef noodle				2	2 med. fat	½	320
Cheeseburger macaroni				1½	2 med. fat	1	360
Tuna Helper (one portion, prepared as directed)							
Creamy noodles 'n tuna				2	1	1½	280
Noodles, cheese sauce 'n tuna				1½	1	½	230
Country dumplings 'n tuna				2	1	½	230

GENERAL MILLS

	Serving size ½ can (prepared ounces)	Food Exchanges					
		Milk	Vege-table	Bread	Lean Meat	Fat	Calories
Casseroles and Side Dishes (one portion prepared as directed)							
Noodles almondine		¼		1½		2½	240
Noodles romanoff		½		1		2½	230
Macaroni and cheese		½		2		2½	310
Noodles stroganoff		½		1½		2	230
Baking Mix							
Bisquick	2 oz. mix (about ½ cup)			2½		1½	240
Ready-to-eat Cereals							
Cheerios				1½			
Corn total				1½			

	Serving size ½ can (prepared ounces)	Food Exchanges					Calories
		Milk	Vege-table	Bread	Lean Meat	Fat	
Country corn flakes				1½			
Kix				1½			
Total				1½			
Wheaties				1½			
Pancake Mixes (for three 4″ pancakes prepared as directed)							
Betty Crocker buttermilk pancake mix				2		2	
Betty Crocker complete buttermilk pancake mix				2½		½	
CAMPBELL'S CANNED PRODUCTS							
Barbecue beans	4			2			140
Beans & franks	4			1	1	1	185

	Serving size ½ can (prepared ounces)	Milk	Vege-table	Bread	Lean Meat	Fat	Calories
							Food Exchanges
Home style beans	4			2			150
Old fashioned beans	4			2			145
Pork & beans	4			2			130
Tomato juice	6		1				35
"V-8" cocktail vegetable juice	6		1				35
"V-8" spicy hot cocktail vegetable juice	6		1				35
FRANCO-AMERICAN PRODUCTS							
Beef ravioli in meat sauce	7½		1	2	1		220
Beef RavioliO's in meat sauce	7½		1	2	1		220
Beefy mac—macaroni 'n beef in tomato sauce	7½		1	1½	1	1	220
Elbow macaroni & cheese	7¼			2	1	1	180
Macaroni & cheese	7¼			2	1	1	180
Meatball mac—macaroni & meatballs in tomato sauce	7½		1	1½	1	1	220

	Serving size ½ can (prepared ounces)	Food Exchanges						Calories
		Milk	Vege-table	Bread	Lean Meat	Fat		
Rotini in tomato sauce	7½		1	2		1		200
Rotini & meatballs in tomato sauce	7¼		1	1½	1	1		230
Spaghetti in meat sauce	7¾		1	1	1	1½		220
Spaghetti in tomato sauce with cheese	7½		1	2				170
Spaghetti with meatballs in tomato sauce	7¼		1	1	1	1		210
SpaghettiO's in tomato and cheese sauce	7½			2				160
SpaghettiO's with little meatballs in tomato sauce	7½		1	1	1	1		210
SpaghettiO's with sliced franks in tomato sauce	7½		1	1½		2		210
Beef gravy	2 oz.					1		30
Brown gravy with onions	2 oz.					1		25
Chicken gravy	2 oz.					1		50
Chicken giblet gravy	2 oz.					1		35
Mushroom gravy	2 oz.					1		35

| | Serving size ½ can (prepared ounces) | Food Exchanges | | | | | |
		Milk	Vege-table	Bread	Lean Meat	Fat	Calories
SWANSON CANNED PRODUCTS							
Boned chicken	2½ oz.				2		110
Boned turkey	2½ oz.				2		110
Chicken spread	1 oz.				1		70
Chunk white chicken	2½				2		110
Beef broth	6¾			Free			
Chicken broth	6¾			Free			
Beef stew	7½		1	1	1	1	190
Chicken stew	7½		1	1	1	1	180
Chicken à la king	5¼			½	2	1	190
Chicken and dumplings	7½			1	2	1	230
Chili con carne with beans	7¾			2	2	1½	310

SWANSON FROZEN PRODUCTS

	Serving size ½ can (prepared ounces)	Milk	Food Exchanges Vege- table	Bread	Lean Meat	Fat	Calories
Meat Pies	one com- plete pie (ounces)						
Beef	8			3	1	4	430
Chicken	8			3	1	4	450
Turkey	8			3	1	4	450
Macaroni & cheese	7			2	1	1	230
Hungry-Man Meat Pies							
Beef	16		1	4	3	7	770
Chicken	16		1	4	3	7	780
Sirloin burger	16		1	4	3	7	800
Turkey	16		1	4	3	7	790

| | Serving size ½ can (prepared ounces) | Food Exchanges | | | | | |
		Milk	Vege-table	Bread	Lean Meat	Fat	Calories
Entrées	one complete entrée (ounces)						
Chicken nibbles with french fries	6			2	2	3	370
English style (fish 'n' chips)	5			1½	2	2	290
French toast with sausage	4½			2	2	1	300
Fried chicken with whipped potatoes	7			2	2	2	360
Gravy & sliced beef with whipped potatoes	8			1½	1	1	190
Meatballs with brown gravy & whipped potatoes	9¼			2	2	2	330
Meatloaf with tomato sauce & whipped potatoes	9			2	2	2	330
Pancakes & sausages	6			3	1	5	500
Salisbury steak with crinkle-cut potatoes	5½			2	2	3	370
Spaghetti with breaded veal	8¼			2	1	2	290
Turkey/gravy/dressing with whipped potatoes	8¾			2	2		260

	Serving size ½ can (prepared ounces)	Food Exchanges					Calories
		Milk	Vege-table	Bread	Lean Meat	Fat	
Hungry-Man Entrées							
Barbecue flavored fried chicken with whipped potatoes	12			3	4	3	550
Fried chicken with whipped potatoes	12			2	5	4	620
Lasagna & garlic roll	12¾			3	2	5	540
Salisbury steak with crinkle-cut potatoes	12½			2½	4	5	640
Sliced beef with whipped potatoes	12¼			1½	4		330
Turkey/gravy/dressing with whipped potatoes	13¼			2	4		380

These recommendations have been developed by Campbell Soup Company, based on the 1976 Standard Exchange Units set forth by the American Dietetic Association and American Diabetes Association, Inc., and are intended as a guide in diabetic meal planning. The nutritive compositions of Campbell products is available upon request.

DIABETIC FOOD EXCHANGE LIST FOR McDONALD'S RESTAURANTS

| | Food Exchanges | | | | | |
	Milk	Vege-table	Bread	Lean Meat	Fat	Calories
Hamburger			2	2	1	331
Cheeseburger			2	2	2	376
*Quarter Pounder (weight before cooking ¼ lb.)			2	3	2	449
*Quarter Pounder with cheese			2½	4	3	602
Big Mac			2½	3	4	574
Fillet-O-Fish			2½	2	3	529
French fries (regular order)			2		2	230
*Egg McMuffin			2	2	3	421
Scrambled egg				2		146
English muffin, buttered			2		1	185
*Hot cakes, buttered, with syrup			6		1	465
Pork sausage				1	2	190
*Apple pie			2		4	320
*Cherry pie			2		3	275

	Milk	Vege-table	Bread	Lean Meat	Fat	Calories
				Food Exchanges		
*Chocolate shake	1		2½		2	435
*Strawberry shake	1		2½		2	435
*Vanilla shake	1		3		2	470
Milk 8 oz.	1				2	260
Orange juice 6 oz.		1 fruit				60
Tomato juice 6 oz.		1				37
*Coca-Cola 11 oz.		3 fruit				120
Sugar-free soft drinks (where available)						

*Persons with diabetes are discouraged from eating these items. The carbohydrate in these items is derived chiefly from sugar. This carbohydrate is quickly absorbed, resulting in an abrupt peaking of the blood sugar.

For further information, contact Denis Detzel or Linda Gelberd, Corporate Responsibility Group, McDonald's Corp., One McDonald Plaza, Oak Brook, IL 60521.

Diabetic Exchange Lists available from the American Diabetes Association, 2 Park Avenue, New York, NY 10016. Exchange List Values determined by the American Diabetes Association, Greater Chicago and Northern Illinois Affiliate, Inc.

FOOD BUYING GUIDE FOR FRUITS AND VEGETABLES

The following chart is from the August 1979 "National Consumer Buying Alert," a publication of The White House, Office of Special Assistant for Consumer Affairs.

Storage and cooking properly can maximize your nutrient intake from both fruit and vegetables. The chart lists the nutrients contained in common fruit and vegetables and gives tips for storing, including the lapse of time before eating quality is affected. Serving yield per pound or piece(s) is also provided. As you will note in our Fruit and Vegetable Exchange Lists, one serving usually equals approximately ½ cup, 1 medium, or 2 small fruits.

Use as little water or liquid as possible to better preserve the nutrients in cooking. (Steaming vegetables on a rack with water under the rack is a fine way to retain food values.) Another nutrient-preserving way to cook potatoes and other root vegetables that are high in water content is in a microwave oven without water.

Product	Nutrients*	Storage Tips	For Best Eating Quality Use Within**	Servings per Unit***
Fresh Vegetables				
Asparagus	Vitamins C and A, iron	Refrigerate in crisper or in plastic bags.	2 or 3 days	2 or 3 per pound
Beans, lima	Iron, B vitamins, fiber	Store uncovered in pods in refrigerator.	3 to 5 days	2 or 3 per pound
Beans, snap	Iron, fiber	Refrigerate in crisper or in plastic bags.	1 week	5 or 6 per pound

Product	Nutrients*	Storage Tips	For Best Eating Quality Use Within**	Servings per Unit***
Beets	Fiber	Refrigerate in crisper or in plastic bags; remove tops before storing.	2 weeks	3 or 4 per pound
Broccoli	Vitamin A, B vitamins, vitamin C, iron, magnesium, fiber	Refrigerate in crisper or in plastic bags.	3 to 5 days	5 or 6 per pound
Brussels sprouts	Vitamin C, B vitamins, iron, magnesium, fiber	Refrigerate in crisper or in plastic bags.	3 to 5 days	5 or 6 per pound
Cabbage	Vitamin C, fiber	Refrigerate in crisper or in plastic bags.	1 or 2 weeks	11 or 12 per pound (shredded) 4 to 5 per pound (cooked)
Carrots	Vitamin A, fiber	Refrigerate in crisper or in plastic bags; remove tops before storing.	2 weeks	5 or 6 per pound
Cauliflower	Vitamin C, fiber	Refrigerate in crisper or in plastic bags.	1 week	6 (raw) 5 (cooked)

Product	Nutrients*	Storage Tips	For Best Eating Quality Use Within**	Servings per Unit***
Celery	Fiber	Refrigerate in crisper or in plastic bags; dry thoroughly if washed before storing.	1 week	3 (raw) 6 to 7 (cooked)
Corn	Fiber	Store unhusked and uncovered in refrigerator.	1 or 2 days	1 per ear
Cucumbers	—	Refrigerate in crisper or in plastic bags.	1 week	5
Greens (kale, collards, etc.)	Vitamin A, B vitamins, vitamin C, calcim, iron, magnesium, fiber	Refrigerate in crisper or in plastic bags; dry thoroughly if washed before storing.	3 to 5 days	6
Lettuce	—	Refrigerate in crisper or in plastic bags; dry thoroughly if washed before storing.	1 week	6 to 8 cups shredded per pound
Mushrooms	Fiber	Refrigerate in crisper or in plastic bags.	1 or 2 days	9 (raw) 4 (cooked)

Product	Nutrients*	Storage Tips	For Best Eating Quality Use Within**	Servings per Unit***
Okra	Vitamin C, fiber	Refrigerate in crisper or in plastic bags.	3 to 5 days	5
Onions, green	—	Refrigerate in crisper or in plastic bags.	3 to 5 days	4 to 6 per bunch
Onions	—	Store in cool (60°F), dry place.	Several months	3 to 4—cooked
Peas, green (in pods)	B vitamins, iron, fiber	Store uncovered in pods in refrigerator.	3 to 5 days	2
Potatoes	Vitamin C, B vitamins, fiber	Store in dry dark place (45°–50°F). Note that potatoes will lose vitamin C gradually over a period of several months	Several months	3 or 4 per pound
Radishes	—	Refrigerate in crisper or in plastic bags; remove tops before storing.	2 weeks	6

Product	Nutrients*	Storage Tips	For Best Eating Quality Use Within**	Servings per Unit***
Spinach	Vitamin A, B vitamins, vitamin C, calcium, iron, magnesium, fiber	Refrigerate in crisper or in plastic bags; dry thoroughly if washed before storing.	3 to 5 days	6
Squash, summer	Fiber, vitamin A	Refrigerate in crisper or in plastic bags.	3 to 5 days	4
Fresh Fruits				
Apples	Fiber	Wash and dry, then refrigerate.	Few weeks	3 or 4 per pound
Apricots	Vitamin A, fiber	Wash and dry, then refrigerate.	3 to 5 days	5 to 6 per pound
Bananas	B vitamins, magnesium, fiber	Ripen at room temperature. Store in refrigerator. Skin will darken, but flesh will remain flavorful and firm.	3 to 5 days	3 or 4 per pound

Product	Nutrients*	Storage Tips	For Best Eating Quality Use Within**	Servings per Unit***
Blueberries	Iron, fiber	Do not wash before storing. Refrigerate—leave on stems and store loosely in shallow container so air can circulate and bottom fruits are not crushed.	3 to 5 days	3 or 4 per pint
Cherries	Vitamin C	Do not wash before storing. Refrigerate—leave on stems and store loosely in shallow container so air can circulate and bottom fruits are not crushed.	1 or 2 days	5 or 6 per pound
Grapefruit	Vitamin C	Store at cool room temperature	2 weeks	2 per fruit
Grapes	Vitamin C	Refrigerate—will not ripen further after picking, so choose ripe fruit.	3 to 5 days	5 to 6 per pound

Product	Nutrients*	Storage Tips	For Best Eating Quality Use Within**	Servings per Unit***
Nectarines	Vitamin A, fiber	Wash and dry, then refrigerate.	3 to 5 days	3 or 4 per pound
Oranges	Vitamin C, fiber	Store at cool room temperature.	2 weeks	3 to 4 per pound
Peaches	Vitamin A, fiber	Wash and dry, then refrigerate.	3 to 5 days	3 or 4 per pound
Pears	Fiber	Wash and dry, then refrigerate.	3 to 5 days	3 to 4 per pound
Pineapple	—	Wash and dry, then refrigerate. Will not ripen further after picking, so select ripe fruit.	1 to 2 days	6 to 8 per fruit
Plums	Vitamin C, fiber	Wash and dry, then refrigerate.	3 to 5 days	3 to 4 per pound
Raspberries	Vitamin C, iron, fiber	Do not wash before storing. Refrigerate—leave on stems and store loosely in shallow container so air can circulate and bottom fruits are not crushed.	1 or 2 days	4 to 5 per pint

Product	Nutrients*	Storage Tips	For Best Eating Quality Use Within**	Servings per Unit***
Strawberries	Vitamin C, iron, fiber	Do not wash before storing. Refrigerate—leave on stems and store loosely in shallow container so air can circulate and bottom fruits are not crushed.	1 or 2 days	3 to 4 per pint
Watermelon	Vitamin C	Wash and dry, then refrigerate. Will not ripen further after picking, so shop for ripe fruit.	3 to 5 days	10 or more depending on size

*Most fruits and vegetables contain no cholesterol and little or no fat. Most vegetables provide less than 50 calories per serving. Starchy vegetables—corn, lima beans, peas, and potatoes—provide less than 100 calories per serving. (See Fruits and Vegetables Lists for accurate amounts.)

**Storage time is longer for unripened fruits and vegetables, but once ripe, these numbers apply.

***One serving equals approximately ½ cup, 1 medium-sized fruit, 2 small fruits, or ½ banana.

RECOMMENDED DIETARY ALLOWANCES, REVISED 1980*

Designed for the maintenance of good nutrition of practically all healthy people in the United States of America. Food and Nutrition Board, National Academy of Sciences–National Research Council.

age and sex group	weight kg.	weight lb.	height cm.	height in.	protein gm	fat-soluble vitamins: vitamin A μg. R.E.†	vitamin D μg‡	vitamin E mg. α T.E.#	water-soluble vitamins: vitamin C mg.	thiamin mg.	riboflavin mg.	niacin mg. N.E.¶	B_6 mg.	vitamin folacin μg.‖	vitamin B_{12} μg.	minerals: calcium mg.	phosphorus mg.	magnesium mg.	iron mg.	zinc mg.	iodine μg.
infants																					
0.0–0.5 yr.	6	13	60	24	kg.×2.2	420	10	3	35	0.3	0.4	6	0.3	30	0.5**	360	240	50	10	3	40
0.5–1.0 yr.	9	20	71	28	kg.×2.0	400	10	4	35	0.5	0.6	8	0.6	45	1.5	540	360	70	15	5	50
children																					
1–3 yr.	13	29	90	35	23	400	10	5	45	0.7	0.8	9	0.9	100	2.0	800	800	150	15	10	70
4–6 yr.	20	44	112	44	30	500	10	6	45	0.9	1.0	11	1.3	200	2.5	800	800	200	10	10	90
7–10 yr.	28	62	132	52	34	700	10	7	45	1.2	1.4	16	1.6	300	3.0	800	800	250	10	10	120
males																					
11–14 yr.	45	99	157	62	45	1,000	10	8	50	1.4	1.6	18	1.8	400	3.0	1,200	1,200	350	18	15	150
15–18 yr.	66	145	176	69	56	1,000	10	10	60	1.4	1.7	18	2.0	400	3.0	1,200	1,200	400	18	15	150
19–22 yr.	70	154	177	70	56	1,000	7.5	10	60	1.5	1.7	19	2.2	400	3.0	800	800	350	10	15	150
23–50 yr.	70	154	178	70	56	1,000	5	10	60	1.4	1.6	18	2.2	400	3.0	800	800	350	10	15	150
51 + yr.	70	154	178	70	56	1,000	5	10	60	1.2	1.4	16	2.2	400	3.0	800	800	350	10	15	150
females																					
11–14 yr.	46	101	157	62	46	800	10	8	50	1.1	1.3	15	1.8	400	3.0	1,200	1,200	300	18	15	150
15–18 yr.	55	120	163	64	46	800	10	8	60	1.1	1.3	14	2.0	400	3.0	1,200	1,200	300	18	15	150
19–22 yr.	55	120	163	64	44	800	7.5	8	60	1.1	1.3	14	2.0	400	3.0	800	800	300	18	15	150
23–50 yr.	55	120	163	64	44	800	5	8	60	1.0	1.2	13	2.0	400	3.0	800	800	300	18	15	150
51 + yr.	55	120	163	64	44	800	5	8	60	1.0	1.2	13	2.0	400	3.0	800	800	300	10	15	150
pregnancy					+30	+200	+5	+2	+20	+0.4	+0.3	+2	+0.6	+400	+1.0	+400	+400	+150	††	+5	+25
lactation					+20	+400	+5	+3	+40	+0.5	+0.5	+5	+0.5	+100	+1.0	+400	+400	+150	††	+10	+50

*The allowances are intended to provide for individual variations among most persons as they live in the United States under usual environmental stresses. Diets should be based on a variety of common foods in order to provide other nutrients for which human requirements have been less well defined. See text for detailed discussion of allowances and of nutrients not tabulated. See preceding table for weights and heights by individual year of age and for suggested average energy intakes.

†Retinol equivalents; 1 retinol equivalent = 1 μg. retinol or 6 μg. β-carotene. See text for calculation of vitamin activity of diets as retinol equivalents.

‡As cholecalciferol; 10 μg. cholecalciferol = 400 I.U. vitamin D.

#α-tocopherol equivalents; 1 mg. d-α-tocopherol = 1 α T.E. See text for variation in allowances and calculation of vitamin E activity of the diet as α tocopherol equivalents.

¶ 1 N.E. (niacin equivalent) = 1 mg. niacin or 60 mg. dietary tryptophan.

‖ The folacin allowances refer to dietary sources as determined by Lactobacillus casei assay after treatment with enzymes ("conjugases") to make polyglutamyl forms of the vitamin available to the test organism.

**The RDA for vitamin B_{12} in infants is based on average concentration of the vitamin in human milk. The allowances after weaning are based on energy intake (as recommended by the American Academy of Pediatrics) and consideration of other factors, such as intestinal absorption; see text.

††The increased requirement during pregnancy cannot be met by the iron content of habitual American diets nor by the existing iron stores of many women; therefore, the use of 30 to 60 mg. supplemental iron is recommended. Iron needs during lactation are not substantially different from those of non-pregnant women, but continued supplementation of the mother for two to three months after parturition is advisable in order to replenish iron stores depleted by pregnancy.

Estimated safe and adequate daily dietary intakes of additional selected vitamins and minerals.*

age group	vitamins			trace elements†						electrolytes		
	vitamin K	biotin	pantothenic acid	copper	manganese	fluoride	chromium	selenium	molybdenum	sodium	potassium	chloride
	μg.			mg.								
infants												
0.0-0.5 yr.	12	35	2	0.5-0.7	0.5-0.7	0.1-0.5	0.01-0.04	0.01-0.04	0.03-0.06	115- 350	350- 925	275- 700
0.5-1.0 yr.	10- 20	50	3	0.7-1.0	0.7-1.0	0.2-1.0	0.02-0.06	0.02-0.06	0.04-0.08	250- 750	425-1,275	400-1,200
children and adolescents												
1-3 yr.	15- 30	65	3	1.0-1.5	1.0-1.5	0.5-1.5	0.02-0.08	0.02-0.08	0.05-0.1	325- 975	550-1,650	500-1,500
4-6 yr.	20- 40	85	3-4	1.5-2.0	1.5-2.0	1.0-2.5	0.03-0.12	0.03-0.12	0.06-0.15	450-1,350	775-2,325	700-2,100
7-10 yr.	30- 60	120	4-5	2.0-2.5	2.0-3.0	1.5-2.5	0.05-0.2	0.05-0.2	0.1 -0.3	600-1,800	1,000-3,000	925-2,775
11+ yr.	50-100	100-200	4-7	2.0-3.0	2.5-5.0	1.5-2.5	0.05-0.2	0.05-0.2	0.15-0.5	900-2,700	1,525-4,575	1,400-4,200
adults	70-140	100-200	4-7	2.0-3.0	2.5-5.0	1.5-4.0	0.05-0.2	0.05-0.2	0.15-0.5	1,100-3,300	1,875-5,625	1,700-5,100

*From Recommended Dietary Allowances, Revised 1980, Food and Nutrition Board, National Academy of Sciences—National Research Council. Because there is less information on which to base allowances, these figures are not given in the main table of the RDAs and are provided here in the form of ranges of recommended intakes.
†Since the toxic levels for many trace elements may be only several times usual intakes, the upper levels for the trace elements given in this table should not be habitually exceeded.

PRINTED MATERIAL AVAILABLE

For information, we suggest that you write to the following:

Juvenile Diabetes Foundation
23 East 26th Street
New York, New York 10010

Recommended by the U.S. Department of Health and Human Services, Public Health Service, and the National Institute of Health is a booklet called "How to Cope with Diabetes," prepared by the National Institute of Arthritis, Metabolism, and Digestive Diseases, Bethesda, MD 20014.

You may buy a copy of the booklet "Exchange Lists for Meal Planning" from the American Diabetes Association. This pamphlet contains information about the diabetic diet.

Diabetic cookbooks may be obtained by writing to the following sources:

"Family Cookbook"
American Diabetes Assn., Inc.
2 Park Avenue
New York, NY 10016
    Price: $12.95

"Cookbook for Diabetics"
Edited by Gaynor Maddox
Taplinger Publishing Co., Inc.
200 Park Avenue South
New York, NY 10003
    Price: $2.95

Many drug companies that sell products intended for diabetes offer excellent publications on diabetes free of charge. They will gladly forward information upon request. Among these are:

Ames Company
Division of Miles Labora-
    tories, Inc.
Elkhart, IN 46514

*Guidebook for the Diabetic
    Patient, Mr. Hypo is My
    Friend* (a cartoon book for
    the education of pre-school
    diabetics), and a diabetes
    identification key chain.

DIABETES RESEARCH AND TRAINING CENTERS

Dr. Norman S. Fleischer
Albert Einstein College
    of Medicine
1300 Morris Park Avenue
Bronx, NY 10461
(212) 430-2908

Dr. Charles M. Clark, Jr.
Department of Medicine
Indiana University Medical
    Center
1100 West Michigan Street
Indianapolis, IN 46202
(317) 635-7401 (x2266 or 2267)

Dr. Stefan Fajans
Endocrinology & Metabolism
    Division
University of Michigan
School of Medicine
Ann Arbor, MI 58104
(313) 764-4165, or
    763-5256 (admin.)

Dr. William H. Daughaday
Washington University Dia-
    betes Research & Training
    Center
660 South Euclid
St. Louis, MO 63110
(314) 545-3387

Dr. Arthur H. Rubenstein
Diabetes Research & Training
    Center
University of Chicago
950 East 59th Street
Chicago, IL 60637
(312) 947-5536

Dr. George Cahill
Joslin Diabetes Foundation,
    Inc.
1 Joslin Place
Boston, MA 02215
(617) 732-2541, or
    732-2565 (admin.)

Dr. Oscar Crofford
Diabetes Research & Training
    Center
Vanderbilt University
School of Medicine
Nashville, TN 37232
(615) 322-2197

Dr. Joseph Larner
Diabetes Research & Training
    Center
University of Virginia
Charlottesville, VA 22903
(804) 924-5207, or
    924-5860 (admin.)

DIABETES-ENDOCRINOLOGY RESEARCH CENTERS

Dr. Franz Matschinsky
Diabetes-Endocrinology
    Center
University of Pennsylvania
School of Medicine
Philadelphia, PA 19104
(215) 622-3165

Dr. Daniel Porte, Jr.
Diabetes-Endocrinology
    Center
University of Washington
1131 Fourteenth Avenue South,
    at R8
Seattle, WA 98195
(206) 762-1010 x493

Dr. Daryl K. Granner
Professor of Medicine and
    Biochemistry
Department of Internal
    Medicine
College of Medicine
University of Iowa
Iowa City, IA 52242

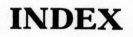

INDEX

INDEX